D1189353

LIBR...
...EDUCATION CENTRE
...OGEND GENERAL

MID GLAMORGAN
COLLEGE OF NURSING AND MIDWIFERY
LIBRARY

CLASS No.......................

BOOK No.....940...................

CLASS No..616..8554.. B✗R

BOOK No......940...................

MID GLAMORGAN
COLLEGE OF NURSING AND MIDWIFERY
LIBRARY

CLASS No. ....

BOOK No. ....

CLASS No. 334

BOOK No. 449

During twenty years working as a speech therapist, both with adults and children, Renée Byrne has observed that the typical stammerer does not exist – each person is an individual. She has also found that the right kind of advice can save a great deal of needless worry – and that people who stammer are often highly articulate and expressive, as becomes evident when some fluency is established and confidence increases.

This book will be useful for anyone concerned with education or child development (including teachers, health visitors and nursery nurses, and for those training to be speech therapists and clinical or educational psychologists), but above all it is intended for adults and teenagers who stammer and for the parents of children with a stammer.

Let's Talk About Stammering

by
RENÉE BYRNE

London
UNWIN PAPERBACKS
Boston   Sydney

616.8554
BYR

First published in Great Britain by George Allen & Unwin 1983
First published by Unwin Paperbacks 1984
This book is copyright under the Berne Convention. No reproduction
without permission. All rights reserved.

UNWIN® PAPERBACKS
40 Museum Street, London WC1A 1LU, UK

Unwin Paperbacks
Park Lane, Hemel Hempstead, Herts HP2 4TE

George Allen & Unwin Australia Pty Ltd,
8 Napier Street, North Sydney, NSW 2060, Australia

© Renée Byrne 1983, 1984

ISBN 0 04 616028 0

LIBRARY
NURSE EDUCATION CENTRE
BRIDGEND GENERAL

Set in Palatino by Bedford Typesetters Ltd
Printed in Great Britain by Guernsey Press Co. Ltd,
Guernsey, Channel Islands

(21.5.97)

Preface

After many years as a speech therapist working with children and adults who stammer, I have become aware that there is a need for a book which gives general information about stammering. This book is written to meet that need. It is intended to help those who stammer, parents, teachers and friends and all who are interested in this subject. It provides answers to the questions most frequently asked: 'What is stammering?' 'What causes stammering?' 'Where can I get help?' 'How can I help myself?' 'How can I help my child?' There is a chapter written about their experiences by people who stammer, and a questionnaire for adults to help them identify their individual difficulties.

For convenience, 'he' is used for the person who stammers and 'she' for parents, teachers, other professionals and colleagues.

I hope that the book will shed light on this perplexing problem and cut through the criss-cross of conflicting evidence, reports and therapies, so that those concerned may be more able to seek help, help themselves or help those around them. For a true understanding, the book should be read in its entirety.

Renée Byrne

Acknowledgments

I would like to thank Peggy Dalton, Rosemarie Hayhow, Celia Levy and Anne Kirk for their valuable comments. I am grateful to Vivien Goodman for typing, re-typing and correcting numerous spelling errors. My thanks are due to my husband, Peter Byrne, for his continuous support. I am indebted to Peter Leek and Michael Radford of George Allen & Unwin for their wise suggestions and amendments. Lastly, I would like to express my gratitude to those many people who stammer from whom I have learnt so much over the years.

LIBRARY
NURSE EDUCATION CENTRE
BRIDGEND GENERAL

Contents

To my Family

LIBRARY
NURSE EDUCATION CENTRE
BRIDGEND GENERAL

Chapter 1

What is Stammering? How Does it Start?

IS THERE A DIFFERENCE BETWEEN STAMMERING AND STUTTERING?

There is no difference between stammering and stuttering. Whether you talk about stammering or stuttering will depend largely on where you live. Stammering is the word most commonly used in the United Kingdom, while stuttering is the term employed in the United States and some other countries.

WHAT IS STAMMERING?

Stammering is speech which is hesitant, stumbling, tense or jerky to the extent that it causes anxiety to the speaker and/or the listener. You may know someone who has this type of speech yet chatters away without any apparent awareness of difficulty. This person may sound like a stammerer, but does not feel like one. Another person may sound far more fluent and yet feels like a stammerer. This is because stammering, in its later stages, is often as much a question of what the stammerer feels as of how he speaks. This is one reason why the condition is complicated. Another is that the very term 'stammering' is confusing. We have only this one word to describe a range of disorders. There is no such thing as 'a stammer', just many different ways in which people speak with a marked lack of fluency. One person may get blocked or stuck on a certain sound or sounds, another may repeat sounds, another may go back and take a run at the difficult word, and yet another may do all these things and many more. When we discuss 'a stammer' it is like discussing 'a broken leg'. Where is the leg broken? In how many places? How severe is the injury? 'A broken leg' is not sufficiently descriptive, and the condition requires considerable investigation.

Equally there is no such person as 'a stammerer'. There is no particular physical or psychological factor which distinguishes a person who stammers from someone who is fluent. To talk about 'a stammerer' tells us nothing about that person except that his speech lacks fluency.

Finally, the term 'stammering' does not differentiate between a small child showing the early signs of the condition and an adult in whom the condition is fully developed. There is a great deal of difference.

Nevertheless, with some reluctance, the terms 'stammering' and 'stammerer' are used in this book as they are generally understood. With the current surge of interest and research in the subject, it is quite possible that more descriptive terms will come into our vocabulary.

HOW DOES IT START?

A young child has to learn many things. He must learn to walk, talk, eat and sit on a potty – all basic acts that are taken for granted, but all requiring complex co-ordination of the brain and body. Just as the child does not suddenly stand up and walk across the room but stumbles, falls and starts again, so fluent speech is not acquired overnight.

There is more to speaking than fluency. Speech involves knowing what we want to say, finding the right words to express our meaning, knowing the right sounds and their correct order to make the words, having adequate breath control to activate the vocal cords in order to produce voice, and co-ordinating all these aspects in smooth, easy speech. It is a complex process. Happily, most children learn the skills of speech spontaneously, and while speech is being learnt other skills, walking, eating and so on, are also being mastered. Some children are quicker in one area, some in another. Very few develop all their skills simultaneously; in fact most tend to spurt in one direction at a time.

Between the ages of 2 and 5 (all ages quoted are approximate) some children show signs of hesitant or disrupted speech and do not have a smooth, easy flow of words. This chapter is written for parents, teachers, doctors, nursery nurses and anyone associated with a child whose fluency is causing concern.

NORMAL DISFLUENCY

There is a tendency to think of fluency and stammering as being poles apart. In the diagram below totally fluent speakers would be at point A and total stammerers at point X.

```
                        O
A ————————————————————————————— X
```

In fact we all hesitate when speaking, insert 'mmm' and 'er', pause unnecessarily, and repeat sounds, syllables and phrases. We get mixed up about what we want to say or cannot choose quickly between two words and so become blocked for a split second. This is quite normal. Totally fluent speech is a fantasy, and so is total stammering. Even an adult with a severe stammer can speak some words fluently and have episodes of fluency.

Stammering and fluency should be considered as a continuum. Some people are nearer to point A, others to point X, but most of us are placed somewhere in between. A person's place is not fixed – there is considerable fluctuation. The division between stammering and fluency at point O is a very fine one. At this point we find people whose speech is not always smooth, flowing and easy. Some of these people consider themselves to be stammerers, others think of themselves as fluent – yet the type of speech produced is quite similar. It is worth noting that although all stammering is disfluent not all disfluency is stammering. Much of what is known as stammering occurs in normal speech and in small children the division between fluency and stammering is even more complex.

Before the age of 5, all children go through a period of disfluency. They are learning to co-ordinate their speech skills and acquire other skills. They stumble, hesitate, pause and try again. This is normal disfluency.

HOW IS NORMAL DISFLUENCY DIFFERENT FROM STAMMERING?

The difference is often subtle. The speech therapist will look for certain indications and try to discover how much of the child's speech is hesitant compared with the amount of fluent speech. She will be looking for the following signs:

The amount of disfluency   A certain amount of disfluency is quite normal in the young child and the therapist will only become concerned if the smooth flow of speech is interrupted very frequently. Since children's speech often fluctuates, she will also wish to know whether or not the child's speech varies from day to day or week to week.

The severity of disfluency   Repetitions, prolongations (holding

on to certain sounds) and even blockages of speech are normal
but if these are accompanied by tension and struggle or by fear
and anxiety that is an indication that the child may be aware of
difficulty and trying to release himself from the unpleasant
sensations of real stammering.

The occurrence of disfluency The therapist will be interested to
know if disfluency occurs mainly in certain situations or with
particular people.

Avoidance behaviour This is a sign that stammering has become
established. The child is now aware of speech difficulties and is
attempting to hide the problem by various tricks and devices. He
may stop speaking during an utterance or use gestures instead of
words. He may look puzzled when asked a simple question,
blush, look away, or start to say a word and then change it for
something different.

HOW DOES STAMMERING DEVELOP?

Often, the early signs are frequent, mild repetitions of sounds
and syllables. Gradually, there is more tension in these repetitions until the tension becomes so strong that speech is literally
'pushed' out and complete stoppages or blocks occur. Once the
child becomes blocked, he also becomes aware that something is
wrong. Slowly, he takes action by increasing tension, by
struggling to release himself from the tension or by somehow
avoiding the moments of disfluency. This may be a common
path.
   There is no conclusive evidence on the development of
stammering, but much well researched and documented
evidence exists which the therapist will consider when trying to
help your child, and I will mention some of the published work.
This summary is by no means comprehensive, but it will reassure
parents that material is available on which to base any advice
which may be given about a child's speech.
   Dr Oliver Bloodstein divides the development of a stammer
into four main phases. Although he emphasises specific
stammering patterns, he does not link them closely with age, but
rather bases them on changes in the speaker's feelings about
speech and about himself as a speaker. For example, in phase 1
there is no feeling of 'being a stammerer' or of 'something being
wrong' – though there may be considerable disfluency, the child
is unaware and unconcerned. He describes the progression of

the stammer in phases 2 and 3 and stresses the changes in feelings and attitudes which are beginning to take place. By phase 4 real fear and anxiety have developed, together with a consciousness of being a stammerer and avoidance behaviour to hide this fact from others.

Dr Charles van Riper talks of four separate developmental tracks or routes which children may follow. He pinpoints different ages when stammering may start and traces development along each of his routes in accordance with different kinds of behaviour related to stammering, general speech and feelings about speech.

The work of Wendell Johnson should also be mentioned. He points out that all children are disfluent, but that adults differ in their evaluation of fluency and in their ability to tolerate mistakes. It is usually the mother who becomes oversensitive to her child's disfluency: she begins to judge it to be a stammer and the child a stammerer.

This judgement may be wrong but, once it is made, adults start to think of the child as a stammerer and the child reacts by becoming aware of his speech and tentative about his ability to speak fluently. Johnson coined the phrase: 'Stuttering starts in the ear of the mother and not in the mouth of the child.'

WHY DOES HE STAMMER?

There is no simple answer. In the light of present knowledge it is almost certain that there is no single reason. A stammer is the result of a combination of different factors, which will vary from individual to individual, and include the following:

A history of stammering in the family   It is known that there is a higher incidence of stammering in certain families. This is not necessarily hereditary, but could be associated with the reaction of members of the family to the normal disfluencies of children.

Some delay in acquiring language and/or articulation   There is evidence that a proportion of children who stammer are slow in mastering the fine, co-ordinating muscular movements needed to articulate, or have had difficulty in learning the words to express themselves. Once these skills are mastered, many children acquire fluency; with others, speech continues to be disfluent.

Considerable emotional stress   This may be due to a single, upsetting incident such as an accident or separation from parents or because there is a constantly stressful atmosphere within the home.

SOME KNOWN FACTS

More boys than girls stammer. The ratios quoted range between 3:1 and 6:1. Stammering in early childhood and throughout its development can fluctuate, moving backwards and forwards. Even when the condition is severe, the symptoms can gradually decrease or suddenly stop. Stammering symptoms are usually worse when the child is anxious, tired, unwell or under stress.

WHY IS ADULT STAMMERING DIFFERENT FROM A CHILD'S?

The outward signs may be the same; it is the feelings and attitude which differ. Take for example Johnny, aged 5, as he goes to school for the first time. He is enjoying himself. He has never heard of a register, never heard a list of names called out. He is interested and, on hearing his own name, answers 'yes' – unaware that he hesitates slightly before doing so. Over the next months, he answers to the register many times. Sometimes he answers easily, sometimes he hesitates or pushes.

Gradually, Johnny becomes aware that he may have difficulty answering the register and so his feelings of unease begin. Slowly he takes avoiding action. Perhaps, after months or years, he coughs before answering, inserts extra sounds or pretends not to hear. The feeling that there is something wrong is developing. Certain words, people or situations must be viewed with suspicion. If the stammer continues to develop, so does the idea of being an inadequate speaker. This is the crucial difference between the young child and the adolescent or adult. The young child may sound the same, but he has not collected sufficient experiences to feel the same.

DOES THE STAMMERING CHILD DIFFER FROM THE FLUENT ONE?

Research shows that there is no psychological or physical difference. The many studies undertaken on this subject tend to show that, in every respect other than speech, the stammering child is normal.

Before discussing prevention and help, it is worth considering the development of a stammer under three headings:

1 *Predisposing factors* may produce a tendency towards stammering. They include a history of stammering in the family; a rather late acquisition of language and/or articulation skills; certain difficulties in co-ordinating the finer muscular movements required for speech.

2 *Precipitating factors* may combine with predisposing influences to tip the balance towards stammering. They include a shock or incident that upsets the child unduly such as illness in the family, starting school, separation from parents, the birth of a new baby, and so on.

3 *Perpetuating factors* affect the situation so that it becomes indefinitely prolonged. These factors are influences on the child which are continuous, such as insistence on very high speech and/or general behaviour standards; a particularly tense or anxious atmosphere in the home; considerable criticism or anger, and so on. One writer talks about the imbalance in the demand/support ratio: there are too many demands on the child in proportion to the help and support provided.

Little can be done about the predisposing factors but, since many children with these influences do not stammer, it is necessary to consider the other factors. Although we cannot shield a child from the shocks and stresses of life – the precipitating factors – we can, through awareness of his distress, help and support him during these episodes. Most crucial, perhaps, are the perpetuating factors, which can cause normal disfluency or early stammering to grow and develop into confirmed stammering.

Examining the precipitating and perpetuating factors will enable us to modify these factors and perhaps *prevent* the development of this disorder.

Chapter 2

Prevention is Always Better Than Cure

Most parents handle episodes of disfluency extremely well. Indeed, Dr Eugene Cooper states that the high rate of recovery amongst child stammerers is probably due to sensible and appropriate management by parents. The following points may serve to clarify certain issues.

The natural reaction to the first signs of a stammer is to try to stop it from becoming worse. This chapter aims to explain why emphasis should be placed not so much on suppressing stammering as on encouraging spontaneous speech free from fear and undue attention. It can take a small child a long time to master the skills of speech – stammering, even if severe, may suddenly stop or gradually decrease. If a child's attention is frequently drawn to his speech, he may become temporarily more fluent, but he will also become anxious, begin to feel that there is something wrong, and form the idea that he is a poor speaker. In order to acquire normal speech, we need to enjoy speaking and find it a pleasurable thing to do. Even a marked stammer can be alleviated, but the problem becomes infinitely more complex once it is linked with feelings of fear and anxiety. For these reasons, it is unwise to interfere directly with a young child's speech.

SPEECH THERAPY

If, over a period of time, you are concerned about your child's speech, ask to be referred to a speech therapist. (Ask your own doctor, a health visitor or the doctor at the maternity and child welfare clinic). If the child seems slow in learning the words to express himself (language) or finds it hard to make the sounds (articulation), it is important to consult a speech therapist. The therapist has the skill to make a clear assessment of the child's whole speech pattern: language, articulation and fluency. She will discuss the findings with you. If the child's speech is found to be adequate, but the disfluency is causing concern, therapist and parents will discuss the best way of managing the situation and helping the child. These discussions may be on the lines suggested in this chapter. The therapist will also learn more about you and your child and this will enable her to produce ideas which are specific to your needs. She will demonstrate speaking and listening skills to clarify these areas, and support you in your task. She will keep in contact with you and, as your fears and anxieties are eased, the problem may disappear. In a few instances, the therapist may decide to see parents and child or to see the child on a regular basis. The sort of help offered will be described in the next chapter. The following advice is offered not as a substitute for speech therapy but as additional information or for those readers who are unable to obtain help.

While it is unwise to interfere directly with the young child's speech itself, it may be possible to change some of the circumstances which perpetuate his difficulties. These include factors associated with the parents or other adults, with the child and with the environment.

PARENTS AND OTHER ADULTS

It is important for parents and other adults concerned about a child's speech to become aware of their own speech pattern. Speech does not develop spontaneously. If abandoned on a desert island, a child will crawl and walk, he will make the babbling sounds of the tiny baby, but he will not acquire language. A French child hears French and learns that language; a German child speaks German. A child will imitate the speech he hears. Consider the following:

How fast do you speak? If you speak too fast, you are giving your child a difficult example. He may try to imitate this fast speech, yet lack the skills to do so. The result can be stammering, tripping over words, or hesitating. Do others in the family speak fast? What chance to express himself has a child got if he is surrounded by this sort of speech?

How urgent is your speech? Urgent and fast speech often go together. However, a feeling of haste may be conveyed even when speech is quite slow. A child will sense this feeling of haste and urgency and may be unwilling to join in if the act of speaking seems unpleasant.

How complex is your speech?   Do you change the subject quite often, sometimes within a single utterance – 'I've got to go to the shops, and Johnny have your drink quickly because Grandma is coming soon'? Do you use complicated words or read difficult books to your child? If so, the child may only understand the gist of what you are saying and never follow the whole message. He will begin to feel that speech is difficult and this will spoil his enjoyment of it.

Communication is the interchange of ideas between the speaker and listener – it is essentially a two-way process. How the listener reacts is important to most of us, but to the young child whose speech is unstable and whose mother is the centre of the world it is crucial. The way you listen is a vital factor in influencing your child's speech:

Interruptions   How much do you interrupt your child with criticism or advice, with comments or questions? If he is constantly interrupted, he will find it difficult to follow a train of thought and impossible to maintain a smooth flow of speech.

Attention   How closely do you attend to your child when he is speaking? It is not a question of stopping other activities and becoming engrossed in the child whenever he speaks, but of the child knowing that you are attending to the message he is trying to convey rather than to the actual words spoken or the way they are spoken. The words we speak do not always reflect our inner thoughts. The child in bed constantly calling for a drink, the toilet, biscuits and so on is not necessarily asking for these items, but probably seeking comfort and attention. Parents often find it helpful to look at their child more frequently when he is speaking and to get down to his level physically rather than standing over him. In this way a child knows he has the adult's attention.

Pleasure and fun   If there are too many occasions when you are irritated or bored when the child speaks and too few when you are pleased and having fun, these feelings will be conveyed to the child. He will become anxious to please with what he is saying or how he is saying it. This can make him over-aware of the act of speaking and inhibit easy, spontaneous talking.

THE CHILD

As a parent, you will know your child, but you may not link

certain characteristics of the child with the way he speaks. It is impossible to categorise children as they grow and change continuously and each is an individual, but some points will provide guidelines on personal characteristics that can influence speech. The placid, quiet child may not need to speak very much, but will do so when he wishes and has something to communicate. He is unlikely to be intimidated by strangers. The active child may be putting most of his energy into physical activity and giving less time to speech. He is often in such a hurry that he hasn't enough time to finish sentences. Just as he stumbles over furniture, so he stumbles over words. The timid, shy child may be unwilling to speak except when familiar with those around him. The curious child will constantly ask why, where and when questions – often not waiting for an answer to one question before asking the next. He can be so over-eager in his quest for knowledge that he stumbles in his haste to obtain more.

THE ENVIRONMENT

Environmental factors are of great importance in a child's development, including speech development.

GENERAL STANDARDS

Do you expect very high standards in manners, behaviour, obedience, and so on? If so, you may be censorious or cross for considerable parts of the day. Perhaps these high standards are based on your own upbringing, or an intense desire to give your child the best start and the best opportunities. This is natural, but the object may be defeated if the child is unable to meet the requirements and so becomes anxious. Anxiety hinders fluency, so it is worth considering the long-term rather than the immediate effects. A young child needs to feel accepted, warm and loved. If he is sensitive, he may be unable to cope with too much criticism, because he fears he is losing the love he craves.

SPEECH STANDARDS

Is a 'high standard' of speech important to you? To some people it is important that those around them speak with an acceptable accent, use a wide range of words, and have a melodious voice and smooth, fluent speech. Others are hardly aware of these aspects and are more interested in other issues. If you believe that the child must speak well for social and educational reasons, are you over-aware of speech and are your standards too high for this particular child? If so, he may also develop an over-awareness of speech and begin to feel inadequate as he finds himself unable to meet your expectations.

FLUENCY

If your speech standards are generally high, fluency and disfluency may assume great significance for you. Undue attention to them will be noted by a child and will eventually have some effect. Both praise of fluency and criticism of disfluency can have adverse results. If the child receives extra attention when disfluent, he may become aware of this and so use his disfluency to gain attention. This is not a conscious decision in a young child but, like other attention-seeking devices, it occurs instinctively and is then reinforced by adult reactions. Conversely, if the child is praised for fluency, he may strive too hard to attain it and begin to use tricks and devices to avoid disfluency and stammering.

General points in management can now be listed:

- Watch your own speech. Shape it towards the model you would like your child to imitate. Reduce speed and urgency. Use the kind of words and the length of utterance suited to the child's level of understanding.
- Be careful how you listen. Limit the number of interruptions and critical remarks. Attend to what the child is attempting to convey rather than the way he talks.
- Do not interfere directly with the child's speech by putting pressure on him to speak or perform in front of visitors. Do not teach him tricks to facilitate fluency, such as 'Take a deep breath', 'Slow down' or 'Say that word again'. Do not teach him complicated words that he does not understand and cannot say easily. As far as possible, allow him to speak freely and when he wishes.
- Think of him as a whole, growing person and not as an inadequate speaking machine. There must be many things he does well. Consider the positive value of praise as against the negative connotations of criticism.
- Speech is more difficult for a child who is ill, anxious, or overexcited. Be aware of this and watchful for such occasions. When they occur, do not pressurise the child to speak.
- Do not call the child a stammerer. Once a label is attached, it is difficult to escape. It is common for children to get labelled

at school – 'He is no good at sports', 'She can't do maths', and so on. Once labelled, a child begins to accept the adult's evaluation and doubts his own ability. This makes the child tense and anxious about his future performance until it becomes impossible to unravel whether there is a real inability or whether the feelings of anxiety have become so acute that ability is smothered. Labelling a child as a stammerer may well aggravate the problem.

- If your child shows real distress when struggling with a word he cannot say, try one of the following: (a) Calmly suggest the word to him so that he can continue without fuss. (b) Assure him that everyone sometimes has difficulty with what they want to say and that it is nothing to worry about. (c) Distract his attention towards an activity which he enjoys.

This is important advice. If it is followed, you may note a reduction in your child's disfluency and in his struggle to achieve fluency. If you consider the time has come for a more concentrated effort, try the following eleven-day programme. Ideally, if mother and father can discuss this plan and work at it together, it will be more interesting for them and possibly more effective for the child. However, if father is rarely at home or reluctant to participate or if you are a one-parent family, the programme will also be helpful if the mother carries it out by herself, perhaps discussing certain aspects with her husband or other adults in close contact with her child. We all differ in how we wish to bring up our children. If you dislike the idea of a programme, then it may be worthwhile to read it and take from it what you feel will be useful for you and your child, incorporating these aspects into your life on a more flexible basis. For parents who like the idea of specific goals, I must emphasise that this is a general programme and is not meant to be followed rigidly so that it becomes a tedious chore. The programme is intended as a framework and if some points don't apply to you they should be omitted. Conversely, you may wish to spend several days on one or other of the aspects mentioned.

The purpose of the programme is to make changes around your child in order to increase his fluency and enjoyment of speaking.

DAYS 1–3

Become aware of your own speech

Concentrate on the speed and urgency of your own speech. Try to vary the speed and thus increase your awareness of the speed at which you are speaking. Practise by talking to yourself. Say a few sentences as fast as you can, a few as slowly as you can, a few at your ordinary rate. Can you vary the pace according to circumstances? With elderly people and young children it is often necessary to speak at a slowish rate. Try these variations throughout the day and make some decisions about your speech. Become aware of any inner urgency and haste. Do you often feel rushed and bothered? Do you convey these feelings when speaking?

DAY 2

Concentrate on the sort of words you use and how much you say at one time. Are you using adult phrases and words? Do you often say a great deal at one time? Does your child understand most of what you say or should your speech be more simple?

DAY 3

In view of your findings on the previous two days, adapt your speech in the direction that would help your child. Work at keeping it slow enough, calm enough and simple enough for his level of understanding and his needs.

DAYS 4–7

DAY 4

Become aware of yourself as a listener

Concentrate on interruptions. Perhaps you hardly ever interrupt the child. Perhaps you, other children or adults constantly interrupt him in mid-sentence. Collect information on this during the day.

DAY 5

How closely do you attend and listen to your child when he is talking? Is your reply in keeping with his message? How often during the day are you too busy or tired to really bother with his chatter?
Collect information on this area.

DAY 6

How much fun do you have with your child? How many laughs?

How many cuddles? How often do you express praise or pleasure?
The knowledge gained may surprise you. Many people love their
children deeply and are intensely proud of them, yet express
these emotions rarely in the rush and worry of everyday living.

DAY 7

In view of your findings, make a few changes. Do not do anything
dramatic or the child may be confused at the change in your
behaviour. Just occasionally make slight changes that you feel
are indicated.

DAY 8

Think about the child. Not just about your duty in teaching him
to become the sort of adult you would wish, but as a growing
human being who is trying to make sense of a world that is still
strange and confusing. How does he behave at the moment?
Does he chatter away regardless of whether he makes sense,
knows the words or is fluent – just for the fun of experimenting
with speech? Does he take things more slowly and talk only
when he knows what he wants to say and has an attentive
listener? Is he usually in a hurry, rushing from toy to toy and
never staying with one activity for long? Or does he become
unhappy if an activity in which he is engaged has to be changed?
He is your own special and individual child, and it will help you
to know how he is setting about coping with the world around
him.

DAY 9

In view of your findings of the previous day, allow the child to
continue along his own path a little more. There will be times
when you must intervene because the child's behaviour is dis-
ruptive to the rest of the household or dangerous to himself. You
may find times when you can allow him to pursue his path
without interference for longer than you might have done previously. It is essential to say 'Don't go near the fire'; it may be less
necessary to say 'You've been playing with that car for ages, play
with the train or bricks instead.'

DAY 10

How often do you think about the child's fluency or disfluency
during the day? If very often, concentrate instead on the things

he does well and praise him for these. Smooth speech becomes less important as attention is focused on the whole child instead of specific speech characteristics.

DAY 11

You have now completed ten days of taking a close look at the factors which may perpetuate your child's disfluency. Whatever you have discovered, start by congratulating yourself on carrying out this programme. It is not easy. Then evaluate the situation. Are there changes that should and can be made? Can they be made one step at a time and can you maintain them? Set yourself some definite tasks and aims for the future.

After a period of a few weeks, during which you will gain further understanding of the needs of your child, his disfluency may decrease or disappear. Don't let up. Continue with the plan you have made for yourself, and check the main points to ensure there has been no slide back to the old ways.

OTHER CHILDREN AND ADULTS ROUND THE CHILD

Obviously other members of the household are extremely important. If it is possible, explain the child's needs to grand-parents, aunts and friends and enlist their help. It may not always be possible. Other children often take their cue from parents. If they are old enough, some explanation can be given. Fluency and stammering need not necessarily be mentioned in this explanation. It can be a matter of stating that Johnny is still very young and cannot understand clearly when everyone talks at once, or speaks very fast and gives him no chance to talk.

If there is considerable rivalry between the children or they are very young, this may not be advisable. However, if the person nearest to the child modifies her own behaviour, this will have a marked effect. Extra help from those around is the ideal, but it cannot always be achieved.

NURSERY SCHOOL

If your child is attending nursery school, it is a good idea to discuss his speech with the nurse or teacher. She will be able to tell you about your child while he is at school and you can discover whether or not she is concerned about the child's speech. It is important that the school knows that there should be no direct interference with the child's speech, and about how you intend to manage the situation. In this way, you and the school can work together along the same lines. There may be a speech therapist attending the school and then her advice can be obtained.

Chapter 3

The Schoolchild

Round about the age of 5 most children start formal schooling and this is a big change in their lives. It may be the first occasion when home, mother, brothers and sisters are left for any length of time. There are many changes and many new things to learn – a new routine, the beginning of school lessons, becoming accustomed to other children and adults. Most children look forward to starting school and enjoy every moment from their first day. For a few this is an upsetting and unsettling time. The child who lacks the skill of fluent speech can have this speech affected for good or ill depending on his reactions to the start of school life.

Repetitions, prolongations and other speech disruptions may occur more frequently and become more severe temporarily on entering school; or this may be a long-term change. Conversely, some children's speech shows a marked improvement at this time and this improvement is often maintained. Some show considerable variations – stammering may occur at school and not at home or vice versa. With other children, the first signs of stammering are observed when they start school; it may happen when they learn to read.

The continuum from fluency to real stammering was discussed in Chapter 1. The schoolchild can be at any point on this continuum and, since the condition often fluctuates, he can move along the line – backwards and forwards. There is no fixed link between age and the degree of stammering, though it is supposed that the younger the child the less severe his stammer. This is often true, but most therapists have encountered children as young as 3 or 4 who showed signs of quite severe stammering and considerable frustration when speaking. Much older children can be seen in the early stages of the condition. For this reason, this chapter will not be divided according to age groups but according to the kind of fluency disorder. However, management and treatment will depend on the child's age and general maturity.

The term 'stammering' will be used more frequently at this point for the sake of clarity. This is not to imply that the child is now well on the path of confirmed stammering. Far from it –

many children will stop stammering spontaneously or with a little help from therapist, teachers and parents.

Stammering and lack of fluency can cause considerable concern to adults because the disorder is always changing. It can take many forms, appear in cycles, occur in some situations and not others, when talking to certain people and not others. No categorisation can be truly comprehensive or accurate. A measurement of the speech pattern recorded in a clinic on Monday morning may differ vastly from measurement taken in the home on Monday afternoon. There are methods of measuring stammering according to the amount of disfluency in a given period of time, the type of disfluency, the speed of speech, and so on. The speech cannot be measured at all hours in all situations and so no measure will give a comprehensive picture. As stammering progresses, the feelings of fear, anxiety and lack of self-confidence also grow. These cannot be measured accurately, but certain signs and certain patterns of behaviour will give indications of the child's inner state. Much will depend on the clear reports of parents and teachers and, with an older child, on his own reports. The following classification is intended to give information and is not to be taken as a hard-and-fast categorisation. Children do not fit easily under headings.

THE BORDERLINE STAMMERER

This difficulty is generally seen in younger children of about 3–7. Any or all of the speech difficulties that we call stammering may occur – repetitions, prolongations and hard blockings, when the sound or word gets totally stuck. With the borderline stammerer, these difficulties do not happen very often and sometimes occur only when the child is excited, tired or very eager to talk. Alternatively, the child may have frequent repetitions such as 'Mu–mu–mu–mummy' or 'Will– will– will you come here?' Yet these repetitions are so mild that the flow of smooth speech is hardly interrupted and communication is only slightly impaired. The child himself seems unconcerned. With these children, the difficulty seems so fluctuating, infrequent or mild that adults are uncertain whether there is anything to worry about. This uncertainty may be heightened by conflicting advice received from neighbours, relatives and friends. At one extreme, you may be told: 'You must do something or Johnny will become a stammerer.' This remark is frequently accompanied by the sort of expression which implies many unspoken thoughts – If Johnny becomes a stammerer it will be your fault; it will be a disaster; I wouldn't allow it; and so on. At the opposite extreme comes the advice: 'Don't do anything. Ignore the whole thing. *I* should know because my son/friend/brother had just the same speech. We ignored it and he's fine.' Who is right? What is to be done?

THE BEGINNING STAMMERER

The child has moved along the continuum and is now definitely stammering. This stage may be seen at any age from about 5 until school-leaving. It differs from the borderline stage in some or all of the following ways:

- A certain pattern is emerging and the stammer is no longer totally random. There may be a problem with certain sounds and not with others: for example, *T*ommy, *t*able, and *t*eapot present difficulty while *S*ally, *s*un and *s*ausage do not. The problem may become associated with certain situations: the child can go to the chemist and ask for anything, but often has trouble when asking for a book at the library. The child may have difficulty when talking to certain people and not others.
- The fluctuations are less and the episodes of stammering more consistent and frequent.
- Although the child is aware of the stammer when it occurs there is little concern or anxiety. There may be momentary frustration or annoyance when the stammer is severe.
- There may be signs of tension and struggle when speaking.
- When speech is interrupted, the child occasionally appears helpless and unable to go on speaking.

Dr Dean Williams states: 'Children vary markedly in the ways they react toward stuttering. One child may profess little concern about the way he talks. He is outgoing and mixes easily with other children and with adults. He speaks, for the most part, spontaneously. He may talk so frequently at home or at school – even though he "stutters" considerably – that parents and teachers are baffled as to how to handle him. Generally, he does not act in a way that stutterers are "supposed" to act. The next child may present the opposite end of the reaction continuum. He is considerably embarrassed by the way he talks. He is afraid to play with other children for fear they will tease him about the way he talks and he grasps every opportunity to be excused from reciting in class.' Dr Williams points out that most children do not conform to either of these extremes, they tend to oscillate between them. They are at a stage of development when their speech, their reactions to others and the reaction of others to them are constantly changing in a random, unstructured way.

THE CONFIRMED STAMMERER

Now we move along the continuum to the child who shows signs of stammering which are a definite problem not only in communication but in his relationship with others and in his evaluation of himself as a person. This stage is different from the previous stage because it is characterised by the child's need to avoid the act of stammering and to hide the difficulty from others. It usually occurs in the older child from about 10 years to school leaving. With the confirmed stammerer, there is definite evidence of tension and struggle and there may be certain associated features, such as closing the eyes, blinking, tensing the hands or facial contortions. The child may seem to hold his breath when blocks occur or attempt to speak while breathing in. Some children may move quite far along the avoidance route and show fewer outward signs of stammering because they have become competent at avoiding the severer episodes.

So, one child may say 'I would lllllllike some b——bread and b——butter', with long prolongation on the word 'like' and hard blocking with considerable struggle to force out the words 'bread' and 'butter'. Another child may not show such severe outward signs because he has learnt to avoid the difficulty by saying 'Can I have some b– some of the loaf and that (pointing to butter).' This may not *sound* so severe to the listener, but it is further along the continuum than the child who is still struggling with the stammer outwardly and does not have the strong urge to hide his difficulty from the rest of the world. It is often difficult for fluent speakers to understand the significance of avoidance behaviour. A full explanation is given in following chapters.

Chapter 4

Speech Therapy for the Schoolchild

Just as fluency may be seen as a continuum, so can speech therapy. The speech therapist does not change her approach radically because the child is in the borderline, beginning or confirmed stage. Her approach is based on a professional judgement of the needs of the child considering his age, his speech, and his feelings about himself and about his speech.

QUESTIONS OFTEN ASKED

If I take my child to a speech therapy clinic will the therapist make him aware that he has a problem and so increase that problem?

The therapist's job is to help the child according to what she sees and hears and according to reports from parents and teachers. If she finds the child is unaware of difficulty, this will be taken into consideration. The therapist will not create awareness where none exists. However, awareness and anxiety are two separate issues, which are not necessarily linked. As a parent, you may be anxious about your child's lack of fluency – while your child is chattering away apparently unconcerned. You make make the assumption that, since the child is unconcerned, he is also unaware. This is by no means so. Many children in the early stages are aware of the stammer when it occurs but are unconcerned. They become interested in what they are saying or in some other activity and their awareness is momentary and fleeting. They are not anxious, because they have no particular feelings about speech in general, about themselves as speakers or about the reactions of listeners. The therapist will consider all aspects in her attempt to prevent the growth of fear and anxiety which are the unpleasant attributes of confirmed stammering.

If the child has to miss school lessons to attend speech therapy, could this make him feel different from other children in his class?

In most instances, therapist and teacher can consult together so that a child missing some time at school is not taken out of important class sessions. The child might feel different if he were the only one to come out of classes; but there are other special activities that children attend and they become accustomed to their classmates missing occasional periods. The child could be worried if he found speech therapy unpleasant. Since the therapist's aim is to create a caring and accepting relationship, it is unlikely that the child will feel singled out – on the contrary, he is often envied and other children ask to join the speech sessions. The general speech activities involved in the early stages would benefit any child and the young child with a stammer may be fortunate to have this opportunity. The child with a confirmed stammering pattern frequently welcomes the chance to have understanding and helpful professional guidance.

There are certain districts in the United Kingdom where holiday courses in groups or individually may be arranged if this is thought advisable so that the school curriculum is not disturbed.

Surely any treatment could make my child worse because the longer the stammer is hidden from him the greater his chance of a cure?

This is a dangerous assumption. The parents' feeling that, if hidden, the difficulty may disappear is not supported by the evidence. True, many children stop stammering suddenly or over a period of time, but the exact reasons for this are not known. Many issues are involved, including good management.

'Hiding' and 'exposing' are extreme concepts suggesting that the therapist will say either 'Hallo, Johnny. You stammer and we will do something about that' or, at the other extreme, 'Hallo, Johnny. I have no idea why you have come to see me because your speech is very good.' There are many possibilities between these extremes and the therapist will exercise her skill and judgement to help your child in the way most appropriate to his needs.

Sometimes parents feel that their child may mislead the therapist. He may well do so, but probably not about his stammer. A child may come into the speech therapy room and

say, 'I've come because I stammer.' The therapist is highly unlikely to accept this statement at face value. She will first ascertain
what the child means – some young children have heard the
words 'stammering' and 'stammer' but have little idea what they
mean. The therapist may ask, 'What do you mean by that? I don't
quite understand.' Answers I have been given include the
following:

> 'Well, it's to do with not being good at reading' – a teacher may
> have commented on the child's speech during a reading lesson.
> The child has few ideas about speech, but is involved in
> learning to read. He interprets the teacher's critical remarks as
> referring to his reading ability and not to his lack of fluency.

> 'I don't know; it's something to do with saying the right
> words' – the child may have been told to stop and say a word
> again on several occasions. He believes this is because he
> chose the wrong word and not because the word was spoken
> with a stammer.

> 'My mum says I'm not *trying* to speak' – the child does not
> understand this remark. His mum makes it when he has just
> finished speaking, so what can she mean?

The therapist will listen and move slowly in evaluating the
situation, making friends with the child and forming plans about
the kind of treatment in the particular instance.

The question is irrelevant with the confirmed stammerer
because he is aware of his stammer.

How long should I wait before asking the speech therapist's advice?

If you are anxious about your child's speech, a therapist should
be consulted. The reasons are as follows:

- The child may be passing through a phase of normal disfluency or may be in the borderline stage when some explanation and reassurance from the therapist may be all that
  is needed to prevent the development of difficulty.
- The earlier a clear assessment of the situation is made, the
  greater the chances of arresting the problem before it becomes
  firmly established.
- There may be good reasons for your concern because the
  child is actually stammering.
- Sooner or later, the anxiety of adults will be noticed by the

child and may contribute to the development of a real stammer. Regardless of whether the child's speech difficulty is trivial or severe, discussions between parents and therapist are important to relieve the parents' anxiety before the child becomes conscious of these feelings.

What does speech therapy involve?

The younger the child, the more vital the part that parents play. With younger children, it is virtually impossible for the therapist to proceed without parental co-operation. Speech is a continuous, moving and living process by which we interact with those around us and express our thoughts, ideas and needs, ask questions and form friendships. The therapist might only see your child for a short period every week and, unless her suggestions can be implemented from week to week within the home, there is little chance of progress being made.

Individual therapy on a once-a-week basis is the most common method in the United Kingdom but in certain parts of the country children may attend in small groups. A group may consist entirely of children who have a stammer. It would meet for about an hour once or twice weekly or, during the holidays, on an intensive basis, for several hours daily for from one to three weeks. Other groups may include children with all types of speech difficulties. The therapist may consider that although the children have differing problems they will work well together and have more scope for enjoyment and for practising general communication activities. With the inevitable chatter that occurs within a group, the therapist may have a better opportunity to hear and assess speech in spontaneous conversation.

Sometimes groups of parents are formed so that ideas and experiences may be exchanged. It helps if a therapist is available to explain particular points and make suggestions.

This book does not describe specific treatments – a therapist will act according to her findings with each individual child. However, the following outline may reassure parents who feel that speech therapy will make their child over-aware of a speech problem that at present does not worry him. The outline is included in order to explain the various stages available to the therapist, from indirect work (no actual therapeutic contact with the child) to direct therapy (working with the child on aspects of his stammer). There are several intermittent stages between indirect and direct therapy and the therapist will take careful account of all the circumstances when deciding the best approach for a particular child.

Indirect therapy

It may be thought sufficient to work with parents and have no regular involvement with the child. The work then might comprise: a) learning the parents' views and opinions about their child in general and about his speech specifically; b) giving parents information about speech and stammering; c) exchanging ideas about the best way to help the child's fluency.

Therapy involving the child but not focused on speech

The child may be seen in a clinic, but activities will not concentrate on speech. Such therapy includes pre-school groups for observation and diagnosis, and play therapy to help the child put his ideas into words and speak freely in a relaxed atmosphere where the therapist can demonstrate easy, comfortable speaking.

Therapy involving the child and aimed at general speech improvement rather than on fluency or stammering

At this level, work in the clinic is focused on speech improvement, but not on either stammering or fluency. The therapist discusses with the child the subject of 'talking' – how we learn to say words, how we talk words into sentences, how we observe what we do and how feelings of being afraid or embarrassed can interfere with all sorts of things that we want to do. Stammering and fluency are not discussed, but reference is made to the difference between 'talking hard' and 'talking easy'. These are the lines advocated by Dr Dean Williams.

Therapy involving the child and directed towards the reduction of stammering

The therapist acknowledges the stammer, the child is taught a certain technique to improve fluency, but emotional issues are not stressed.

Direct therapy with the child focused on aspects of stammering and fluency

The emphasis is on stammering and fluency. The child is helped with his stammer, but there will also be discussions about the feelings and attitudes he has towards speech, stammering, communication and the reaction of listeners when he is speaking.

Many methods are available to the therapist and she may also have certain aids at her disposal. Some clinics have equipment ranging from cassette or even video recording equipment to Delayed Auditory Feedback machines, internal telephones, and all sorts of other gadgetry which makes the child's visit both productive and enjoyable.

How long will my child have to attend speech therapy?

There are no definite rules – the length of time will depend on the therapist's evaluation of each individual child.

My child has the opportunity of seeing an elocution teacher. Would this be helpful?

There is no precise answer. Some children enjoy elocution lessons and, if your child does, lessons may increase his general confidence in speaking but not necessarily increase his fluency. However, if the child is unhappy about elocution lessons they are not advisable as his awareness of difficulty could be increased.

Chapter 5

How Can Parents Help?

It is always advisable to obtain the help of a speech therapist and, if a therapist is already working with you and your child, the information in this chapter will provide a back-up for ideas which are already familiar to you. The chapter is aimed particularly at parents who are unable to obtain therapeutic help. If you are in this position, do not despair – there is much you can do.

The first step in helping your child is to understand what is involved in the production of satisfying speech. The prevention of stammering was discussed in Chapter 2. We are now dealing with the child who is stammering, and more information is given in order to suggest how to proceed.

DEVELOPMENT

The development of speech in terms of its component parts – language, articulation, voice and fluency – has been discussed. Speech develops slowly and in relation to the child's general development, his personality, his family environment and his interests. Speech development is an individual matter and variations between one child and another can be very wide. As adults we forget how we stumbled, hesitated and searched for words when we were acquiring the skills of speech. We may expect too much from our child too soon – particularly if his speech is compared with that of an older brother or sister or a neighbour's child who may be developing on totally different lines. There is a distinction between knowing how to do something and learning how to do it. We may make the assumption that a child *knows* about speech without allowing him to *learn* and make the mistakes which are essential in any learning process.

When your child first began to make the 'bababa' and 'dadada' noises and gurglings of early speech, you were delighted. As time progressed he began to say words and put two words together – 'me go' or 'mummy car'. These words and short sentences were a source of interest; your pleasure continued with each new step taken – not only in speech, but in all areas of his development. It was not until your son was about 3 or older that you began to notice occasional hesitations and repetitions. Perhaps you accepted these as being something that all children experience; perhaps you made a mental note to keep an eye on his speech or perhaps you became worried in case your child was beginning to stammer.

Speech development is one aspect to consider. Another aspect is your reaction to your child's speech. As a baby he was accustomed to many things he said and did being received with joy and praise. This boosted his emerging self-confidence and encouraged him to try to do and say new things. His world was then, and is now, very dependent on your reactions. How do you react when your child hesitates or stammers? How should you react?

COMMUNICATION

It is easy to forget that communication is what speaking is all about. Communication is interaction between two or more people: ideas and thoughts are spoken by one and received by another, who responds in some way. Speech is influenced by the reaction of others participating in the conversation. To take an example: many fluent people know of occasions when they have felt tongue-tied and inadequate whilst speaking. Such a situation may occur in a restaurant when the food served is below standard. When a genuine complaint is made, the icy aloofness of the waiter coupled with the curious glances of other diners causes speech to become hesitant and confused. The speaker knows what to say and how to say it and would have no problem if alone, but the adverse and critical reactions have a direct effect on his actions and feelings and an inadequate speaking performance results. Most people who stammer can speak fluently when by themselves or when singing because true communication is not taking place.

Effective communication does not depend mainly or solely on fluency. This is shown by the fact that some stammerers are interesting communicators while some fluent speakers are ineffectual and dull communicators. Apart from voice, articulation and language, there is the content of what is being said. Regardless of how perfect speech may be, if the subject matter is uninteresting, communication will be ineffective because the listener will become bored and will not participate. If the speaker is insensitive to the needs of the listener and talks incessantly without allowing others to get a word in edgeways or if he talks dogmatically and authoritatively on every and all subjects, communication will be impaired as the listener will become restless or angry and thus a true interchange of ideas cannot take place.

Apart from speech, there are 'non-verbal' areas of communication. Thoughts are not conveyed only through speech. A surprising amount of information is conveyed without words – by behaviour, looks, dress, movement, and so on.

It is essential to consider all the elements that contribute to communication in order to see the role of fluency in its true perspective as a part and not as the whole of this process.

RELATIONSHIPS

We differ from all other animals in possessing true speech. Our speech is infinitely more complex than the simple signals and signs by which other animals communicate. It is through speech that we mainly relate to each other. Obviously, there are different levels of relationship, from deep love to superficial acquaintance, and speech differs accordingly. With those we love and who love us, we are able to express thoughts and emotions – whether these are pleasant or unpleasant – as there is a feeling of safety in the knowledge of being loved. With acquaintances and colleagues, words are often more considered. If our job is at risk, it may be inappropriate to make a loud, challenging statement however right that statement seems because, in this situation, we are not secure.

Some people are highly aware of reactions to their speech; others are more happy-go-lucky and tend to speak out regardless. Some people are intensely private and speak mostly when they have something significant to say; others need to verbalise their thoughts and share experiences through words. We differ. Our children differ. One thing is certain: the safer we feel in the relationships made in early life with parents and immediate family, the easier will be our path in communication and, through communication, in relationships.

Some authorities define stammering as a problem of interpersonal relationships. If relationships within the home are often hesitant, struggling, fragmented and fraught with anxiety, speech may reflect these hesitations, struggles, fragmentations and anxieties. Not all children react through their speech but, for the stammering child, warm, close relationships within the home are of importance. Disturbed relationships can be a perpetuating factor in confirmed stammering; secure relationships can do much to stem its development.

DISCIPLINE

The issue of discipline causes much controversy. How much? How often? Of what kind? You may feel that there is much truth in the dictum 'Spare the rod and spoil the child' or you may be convinced that corporal punishment and verbal reproval would harm the healthy growth of your child. I am in no position to discuss the rights and wrongs of various forms of discipline, but feel it is important to point out their effects on a child who is stammering.

Very strict discipline often goes hand in hand with demanding of your child high standards of general behaviour. If you think you may err on the side of strictness and high standards, ask yourself why. Is it for the sake of your child? Do you believe these standards are essential to his well-being? Is it for your own sake because you find standards lower than your own difficult to tolerate – especially in your home and in your child? Is it for the sake of neighbours? Do you fear their criticism when your child misbehaves?

The answers to these questions may make you more confident in the knowledge that you are pursuing the right path, or you may decide that you could make some changes.

Children vary in their response to corporal punishment and there is a vast difference between beating a child and giving him a short, sharp smack. If a child is frightened, his disfluency will increase. Fear creates tension and tension leads to incoordination of the muscles required to produce smooth, flowing speech. Corporal punishment is not the only thing that can produce fear. Constant critical words – 'No, don't do that', 'You're very naughty', etc., – can also cause fear, the fear of losing love.

A further consideration is the consistency of discipline. Many difficulties arise when discipline varies sharply according to the moods of parents. Perhaps one day Johnny leaves his room in a terrible state and nothing is said, whilst the next day he is threatened with all sorts of punishments if his room is not tidy within five minutes. Or perhaps some punishment has been justifiably imposed and is then retracted. Discipline in the home is linked closely to relationships. If discipline is fair and consistent and functions within the context of loving relationships, the child will accept it. If discipline is too harsh or inconsistent, the child may become confused and uncertain. Feelings of confusion and uncertainty may emerge as confused and uncertain speech.

Dr Zwitman believes that it is helpful if parents differentiate between unintentional and intentional misbehaviour and adapt their discipline accordingly. He defines unintentional misbehaviour as mischief 'without meaning to do so'; intentional misbehaviour is when a child commits an act knowing it to be wrong or wants to do something which cannot be allowed and so cries and argues to get his own way.

PARENTS

One point is sometimes overlooked: parents are human. As parents we cannot know everything; we also have to learn and, while learning, we make mistakes. There are many pressures – financial pressures, pressures at work, in relationships and in the upbringing of children. Parents are bombarded with advice and admonitions and, all too often, blame themselves for everything that goes amiss with their child. Television advertisements show the 'perfect' housewife who manages to clean the house, get the children to bed, entertain important guests with a wonderful meal and look divine throughout. Sometimes the pressures and demands can be too great.

Chapter 6

Some Practical Advice

This chapter provides suggestions and ideas for helping your child. The advice given should be adapted to individual circumstances, priorities and capacities. It is not necessary to follow the suggestions rigidly – far from it. There are many choices in life; the intention is to make the choices relating to your child's speech easier as the issues involved are better understood.

It is difficult for parents to decide when the subject of stammering should first be discussed with their child. In the early stages and with the young child there should be no direct interference with speech or reference to stammering. However, as the child gets older and more aware of difficulty, or the stammer becomes more firmly established, it does become necessary to talk about hesitations in speech and eventually about stammering. Once the child is aware of his stammer and concerned about it, the situation is made worse if stammering becomes a taboo topic that no one is prepared to bring into the open. If stammering is discussed too early, the child may become anxious and confused; if it is discussed too late, the child may have been allowed to live alone with his difficulty and this will increase his developing fears and perplexities.

This is a delicate decision and, in making it, parents should be aware of the issues involved and sensitive to the needs of their child.

How can I help with communication in general?

- Understand all that is involved in communication and make good communication the goal. Stammering and fluency are only one aspect of the whole.
- Consider your own listening and speaking skills.
- Consider the discipline in your home and check whether you are relatively consistent and fair in its application.
- Remember the continuum of stammering and fluency. Total fluency does not exist – all adults and children show disruptions in their speech. Learn to tolerate these disruptions.

How should I react when my child stammers?

Be clear in your aims: react to the whole act of communication and not specifically to stammering or fluency; help him to become a confident speaker, not just a fluent one.

- Do not tell your child to 'stop stammering' – if he could, he would. You will cause confusion because he does not know *how* to stop.
- Do not threaten, become angry or impatient – if the child is made fearful and tense, he may stammer more and no useful purpose is served.
- Do not speak for your child or answer questions on his behalf – this will underline his inability to speak as efficiently and fluently as you do and tend to make him feel shy and embarrassed when he has to speak for himself.
- Do not say 'Speak slowly', 'Say that word again', 'Take a deep breath' or 'Think before you speak'. These admonitions refer directly to the *way* the child is speaking. They interfere with the spontaneity essential for free speech, and also draw attention to speech and increase the awareness of difficulty.
- React in the same way whether the child is fluent or stammering. React to *what* he is saying and not to *how* he is saying it.
- If he is in a hurry, overexcited or tense, you might say 'Keep calm' or 'There is no hurry, we have plenty of time'. This is different from saying 'Speak slowly' or 'Say that word calmly' because there is no direct reference to speech. The reference is to the fact that the child is in a hurry or overexcited – a significant difference when it is felt necessary to give advice.
- Do not praise your child for being fluent – this makes him feel that you like him when fluent and that fluency is 'better' than stammering. As a result, he may strive too hard for fluency and begin to form ideas about how you react differently when he is fluent and when he is stammering. He may base ideas of how others will react on the reactions he gets at home.
- Do not pay extra attention when your child is stammering. Many bright children learn early in life that when they are stammering parents listen more closely. The result? When you want attention it is a good idea to stammer!

I want to do something definite to increase my child's fluency

The best thing you can do is to worry less about fluency. Speech is spontaneous, natural behaviour and constant emphasis on one aspect of it causes over-awareness and spontaneity and naturalness are lost. Think about walking. Probably you hardly ever think about walking, but there may be occasions when you become extremely conscious of this natural act. Perhaps when walking along a platform in front of an audience with all eyes on you, you find that your legs will not move properly. The walk along that platform seems a thousand miles and the more conscious you become of *how* you are walking, the less able you are to co-ordinate movements. So it is with speech. Being over-aware of certain aspects of speech can interfere with its natural production and increase tension – and the vicious circle of anxiety, more anxiety, more tension begins.

While direct emphasis on making your child more fluent is not advisable, indirect help can be most useful. It will assist the child if one or both parents can share with him whatever activities appeal to the family – indoor or outdoor games, visits to places of interest, doing things about the home and so on. In this way, speech occurs spontaneously and without self-consciousness. The child knows that he has your attention because you are doing something together, but speech is not spotlighted, merely part of the activity.

Reading to the younger child slowly and calmly also helps. Often the child will make animal or train noises to illustrate the story or say some of the words in a familiar story while you are reading. Again the focus is on the story and not on how he is speaking, so this is another way to aid fluency indirectly.

The older child or the confirmed stammerer may wish to talk about his speech difficulties as he is now aware of them. Parents should encourage him to say what he wishes. Chapter 8 gives fuller information.

Sometimes my child seems really 'stuck' on a word. He gets upset and I wonder how to help him

What help you might give depends on his age, on the stage he has reached in stammering, and on whether the incidences are isolated or frequent.

- Consider what the child is doing as 'normal speaking under the circumstances' and examine the circumstances in which he becomes so blocked in his speech. Is he particularly tired, excited, bewildered or afraid? Is he speaking under unusual pressure, in front of strangers or on the telephone? Has he become aware that you are worried when he gets 'stuck' in his speech? Has something changed in the family circumstances – a move to a new house, a new baby or an illness? If you find something unusual in the circumstances, try to prevent the occurrence of such events. If this is impossible, support the child when these events happen. He will tend to take his cues from you and, if you react with reassuring acceptance, he will know that nothing very bad is happening because you are quite calm.

- As a general rule, do nothing specifically related to speech. However, you know your child and the circumstances and may feel that there are occasions when direct help is needed. If so, the following are possibilities:

(a) If you are *sure* of the word your child wants to say and on which he is blocked, say the word slowly and easily; then allow him to finish what he wishes to say.

(b) If the child has considerable difficulty in conveying a message, repeat what he has said and then give an answer. The intention is to establish that you understood his message.

EXAMPLE

Child: 'C–c–c–can we go to the p–p–p–pictures on Sssssssaturday?'
Parent: 'Can we go to the pictures on Saturday? I imagine so, but it will depend on whether Mary gets home in time.'

(c) Reassure the child that we all have times when we find it difficult to say exactly what we want, but that these occasions are soon over.

(d) Distract his attention from the difficult speaking situation to an activity which he enjoys.

(e) If you cannot distract him at the time, shift his attention to a pleasant activity as soon as possible after a period of hard stammering.

Michael is 6 years old. During the past couple of months, he has suddenly started to stammer with marked repetitions and complete blockages

This sudden onset of disfluent speech is likely to induce parental anxiety just because of its suddenness and can also cause anger and frustration in Michael. Take your time in evaluating the situation; give him time to stabilise. It may be that some specific event has upset him and so speech has become temporarily disfluent. Your calm acceptance of these incidents will do much to help Michael. It would be wise to discuss the situation with his class teacher and discover whether she has noticed the change in his speaking pattern. She might suggest an event at school that could have triggered off the change. If your anxiety continues, consult a speech therapist.

John is 15 and beginning to think about his future. He has a severe stammer. He gets depressed and angry worrying how he can cope with exams, girls, the future, etc.

- Is it impossible for John to get some therapeutic help? If you live in the United Kingdom and help is not available in your immediate vicinity, contact the College of Speech Therapists or the Association for Stammerers to discover whether there is a centre in a nearby town where professional help can be obtained.
- If no professional help is available, consider the following points:

    How much have you previously talked with John about his stammer? How much do you talk about his future, his interests, his work and his worries? Much will depend on the answers for people vary markedly in their need, experience and ability to share important issues. It is necessary for John to be able to discuss his hopes and fears as well as the specific problems of stammering. By this stage, John is highly aware of his stammer, and the time for keeping silent is long past. Many people reach adulthood without ever having had an opportunity to talk about their speech impediment. A wall of silence is created. Parents, teachers and friends never mention the subject, believing that it is inadvisable to do so. This silence tends to make the stammerer think that his speech is so unpleasant, different or antisocial that no one likes to mention it. There is a feeling of isolation, frustration and bewilderment as neither the stammerer nor those around him dare to break the silence. Avoiding the subject gives it undue importance. An appropriate moment must be found to talk about stammering with John.

Here are some guidelines for such a discussion:

(a) Do not try to tackle the whole subject in one talk. Think in terms of airing the topic over a period of time.
(b) Take into account the need to encourage John to talk about all aspects of his life and future – not only the stammer.

(c)   Do not concentrate on providing answers. Listen to what
        John has to say. He may become very fluent or stammer
        severely. It is vital to listen and let him feel that you have
        adequate time and want to understand.
(d)   Do not ask too many questions but, as far as possible, allow
        John to do the talking.
(e)   Encourage John to talk to you about anything and
        everything whenever he wishes. The best encouragement
        is to become an attentive and supportive listener.

When you have acquired a greater understanding of how John
feels about his stammer, consider the following possibilities and
discuss these with him.

(a)   John could read Chapters 8–13 of this book relating to
        teenagers and adults, the reports of those who stammer and
        advice on helping yourself. If John feels very alone in his
        difficulty, these chapters may help him to realise that there
        are others who share his difficulty and experiences.
(b)   He could write to the Association for Stammerers as it may
        be possible to find a boy or girl of his age who would wish to
        exchange tapes, telephone calls or letters with him.
(c)   He could read the self-help books mentioned at the end of
        this book.
(d)   Together you could review the self-help advice given in
        Chapter 12.

**I have four children and Mark at 12 years is the second youngest.
He stammers quite badly at times but talks much more than the
other children and seems to monopolise conversations**

It seems that Mark is given undue attention by yourself and the
other children because he stammers. This is unhelpful to him as
strangers may not be so considerate and he is not learning about
good communication. Perhaps Mark feels a need to put all his
thoughts into words and is not particularly aware of or bothered
by his stammer. Begin to treat him in the same way as the other
children and, if he has more than his fair share of speaking time,
tell him so. Say firmly: 'Mark, you are chattering on and on; it is
time that you gave Alan a chance.'

**When I am in a hurry and my son starts to stammer I sometimes
feel irritated and cross**

Most parents do get irritated with their children at times and, conversely, the children get irritated with their parents. However, if these feelings are usually linked with episodes of stammering it may help you to consider possible reasons:

You would like your son to speak well at all times   Possibly he does speak well a considerable percentage of the time but you are oversensitive to episodes of stammering. Perhaps you could learn to accept the stammer and begin to see it as just one part of your son at that moment.

You feel irritated at yourself for being cross   Look at it from a different point of view – being cross is inappropriate at the time when your son stammers because he is speaking as well as he can.

You feel under considerable pressure and ruled by your watch   Is it possible to allow yourself a little more time in general and a few extra minutes when listening to your son?

You are in a genuine hurry to keep an appointment   Be honest and tell your son that you have an appointment to keep, but will listen to what he wants to say on your return.

My son has been seeing a speech therapist for some time. He does not improve

There are several issues which should be discussed with the therapist.

- What is meant by improvement? Perhaps improvement to you is related only to fluency whilst the therapist is working on helping your son to speak freely without anxiety. She may feel that specific help with fluency is not needed or that fluency should be tackled at a later stage.
- Perhaps the therapy your son is being offered is not geared sufficiently to his needs and some change in approach could be considered.
- Alternatively, your son may be uninterested because he is mainly unconcerned about his stammer, finding other activities of greater interest.

You, the therapist, and your son, if old enough, should discuss matters so that the situation can be clarified. It may be that those involved are failing to communicate and share information.

Steve aged 4 is stammering quite badly. I went to see the speech therapist and was told that there was nothing to worry about as he was too young to have therapy

Many speech therapists are under intense pressure to see more people than is possible. They are responsible for seeing children with language and articulation difficulties, physically and mentally handicapped people, those who have been involved in accidents affecting their speech, the elderly stroke patient who has lost the ability to speak, and many more. This means that therapists may give priority to those they feel in the greatest need and it is difficult to establish such priorities. Equally, some therapists are more experienced in one field than another. It is likely that the therapist you saw was either under pressure and thought your child could wait a little longer, or she believed that Steve was passing through the stage of normal disfluency so that he was no different from other children and did not require treatment.

There are some possibilities open to you:

- Perhaps Steve was just passing through a phase and is now more fluent so that the situation is beginning to resolve itself.
- Perhaps you are still worried. If possible, see the therapist again and voice your anxiety. Circumstances may have changed; perhaps she can now do something to help.
- On reading this book and others suggested on page 116 you may have begun to work out a course of action to alleviate your anxieties and help Steve.
- If the above do not apply, discuss the situation with your family doctor or contact one of the organisations mentioned at the end of the book for information about speech therapy services in your vicinity or other areas.

English is not our native language. We speak one language at home and the child speaks English at school and elsewhere. Will this increase his stammer?

It might do so. You will be eager for your child to learn his own language for cultural, social and educational reasons. Many children can cope with two or even three languages – others cannot. It must be accepted that, if your child is showing diffi-culty in any area of his speech, it would be easier for him to use one language consistently. It will be difficult for the child who stammers to think in two languages, formulate the words and sounds of two languages and handle the different melodies or intonation patterns of these languages. Since the schoolchild must speak primarily in English, it would be advisable for parents to speak only in English for an agreed period of time and reconsider the situation at the end of this period. Hopefully, the fluency will increase and the other language can gradually be reintroduced.

My husband stammers and my son hears this. He has started to stammer and I think he is imitating his father

There is little indication that a child learns to stammer through imitation, but considerable indication that in families where stammering occurs extra attention is paid to speech behaviour. Often there is special anxiety because the stammering parent is convinced that the son's stammer is entirely his fault. It is difficult to release oneself from feelings of anxiety, but the advice given in this and previous chapters is relevant to the parent who stammers. Perhaps there are certain advantages in your situation. The stammering child in a household where everyone's speech is very fluent may feel at a disadvantage.

In your home, your husband may help to reassure his son that adults do not always speak fluently. If he can demonstrate that it is possible to stammer easily, without fear or undue self-consciousness, then perhaps the child will follow his example and will not develop the fears which lead to confirmed stammering.

I remember a man with a fairly severe stammer who attended group speech therapy sessions and became much more fluent. One morning he arrived and reported with amazement that he had read a story to his 6-year-old daughter the previous night and had felt extraordinarily proud of his controlled and smooth speech. At the end of the story his daughter said 'Speak properly, Daddy.' 'I am speaking very properly,' said father indignantly. 'No, speak like you always do,' said daughter. This episode illustrates that the little girl loved her father warts, stammer and all – it is the total relationship of child and parents that is of importance. The parents' love, care and interest are of infinite value and, compared with these, the stammering speech is of minor significance.

If your husband feels that he is unable to handle his stammer and is highly anxious about it, would he consult a speech therapist for some help? It is never too late. Stammering therapy has greatly improved in recent years so that men of all ages frequently seek help which was not readily available in their younger years.

This chapter gives practical advice for the difficulties most often encountered. But it must be stressed that stammering is a developing and changing disorder. It cannot be too strongly emphasised that, if at first you don't succeed, try, try and keep on trying!

Chapter 7

How Can Teachers Help?

Teachers are often under considerable pressure when confronted by a class of children many of whom have special needs. But, since the teacher plays such an important part in any school-child's life, she can also be a significant influence on a child's stammering pattern. This chapter examines specific and general difficulties which may be encountered in order to make the task of teaching a child who stammers somewhat easier.

Many caring teachers do not know how to handle stammering and resort to trial and error methods which can cause more uncertainty in both teacher and child. These teachers see a child who stammers as a special case and so make him the subject of special attention in one form or another. The child then begins to see himself as special in a negative sense and may have difficulty in competing on equal terms in later life.

One aim predominates in management and it may well be the aim held by many teachers for children in their charge – that each child, while gaining academic knowledge and added skills, also learns a sense of his own self-esteem and self-worth so that he can go out into society and cope with life's rigours and difficulties without the added burden of a chip on his shoulder. Some children do leave school with such a chip on their shoulder because they have not gained the academic goals required by parents and teachers, because they do not feel socially acceptable, because they do not speak fluently, and so on. The child who stammers needs to learn his own self-worth as a human being so that the stammer, whether permanent or temporary, does not cause long-term scarring.

In Chapter 13 one man writes: 'I do not blame my family for my present stammer . . . but I do hold them responsible for pouring in the concrete that set so deep in me.' This concrete is mixed and formed from the attitudes and reactions of parents and teachers. Once feelings of fear and inadequacy have set deep, they are often more damaging to the person than the actual stammer.

Like everyone else, teachers differ in their reaction to disfluent speech. Some may accept stammering as just something which happens and something to handle in much the same way as other children's difficulty with reading or writing. Others find stammering highly embarrassing, particularly if it occurs in front of the whole class and causes delay in the activity being pursued. If you are concerned about a child in your class who stammers, the first step might be to consider your own feelings. Because so much depends on speaker–listener interaction, there is little point in managing the child if you find considerable anxiety in yourself. Many children, particularly in the younger age groups, are not especially worried about their speech and are surprised by the anxiety of teachers and parents over something which seems trivial to the child at that time.

If you are worried when a child stammers, it may be for one of the following reasons:

- You feel uncertain how to handle the situation and it is this uncertainty which causes anxiety.
- You feel that other children may laugh or comment adversely and this would be a tricky situation.
- You feel the child himself may be embarrassed or upset.

I believe we sometimes focus our own adult experiences and concepts on to a child and evaluate his own standpoint wrongly. This is illustrated by Bob, aged 10 years, whom I saw at a speech therapy clinic. He displayed a very strange stammering pattern in that he held on to sounds such as s, sh and w for approximately six seconds, took a breath, held on to the sound again and then said the word. He would say: 'Shshshshshsh – breath – shshould I open the wwwwww – breath – wwindow?' While talking with his parents, I discovered that his father had stammered and did not want his son to follow the same path. When Bob was 9 years old and had stammered with mild but frequent repetitions for some time, his father discussed the matter with him. Since Bob did not seem to understand clearly, a tape recording was made and father pointed out the re–re–re–repetitions in his sp–sp–speech. Some time after this, Bob began to prolong sounds. When Bob came to see me in the clinic, we formed a good rapport as he was a bright child interested in all sorts of things and so it became both possible and useful to ask him: 'Why do you say "should" the way that you do, holding on to the "sh" sound?' Children frequently give logical and clear answers.

Bob explained that he held on to the sound because, after the discussion with his father, he had begun to understand that it was not a good idea to stammer and that stammering meant the repetition of sounds at the beginning of words – he had heard this on the tape recording. Being given no help, he tried hard to stop making these repetitions and ended by prolonging sounds. Elated because he no longer repeated, he could not understand why his father and teacher still said he stammered. Bob had been given a clear explanation and demonstration that stammering= repetitions; so he stopped repeating and no one seemed pleased. With Bob, there had been a lack of appreciation that the evaluations of children and adults differ.

Being aware of the real feelings of a child about his speech is often a big step in coping with your own feelings and making some management decisions. In this context, co-operation and exchange of information between teacher, parents, therapist and, where possible the child himself is the ideal course of action. Each person has much to contribute to discussion: the therapist knows the best way to proceed as far as speech is concerned; the parents know their child, his home environment, his general behaviour within the home and so on; the teacher knows how the child behaves at school, how he relates to adults and peers, how he copes educationally, and when and how he speaks. If therapist or parents are not available, discussion between the other parties is still helpful so that they can gain more information about the child's needs. You cannot make assumptions. If you are anxious about the fluency of a child in your care, it is always advisable to discuss it with the parents; they may or may not be conscious of the difficulty; it may or may not occur within the home; they may or may not favour a particular course of action.

If the parents have been unwilling or unable to seek the help of a speech therapist, perhaps you could persuade them to do so. The school medical officer may well be helpful.

Indications of the child's attitude and feelings can also be gleaned by observation of his behaviour when stammering. Here are some examples:

- Does he blush, avert his eyes and look generally embarrassed? If so, does this behaviour stop once he has said what he wants to say or does he continue to show signs of concern once he has finished speaking? It is important to differentiate between signs of momentary concern and anxiety which continues for some time after the stammering has stopped.
- Does he push through to the end of the utterance, sometimes with quite severe speech blockages, but still pressing onwards? This may indicate that the child is involved with what he is trying to communicate and not with how he is speaking.

- Does he avoid speaking in some way? Perhaps he starts to speak and then stops, looks confused, pretends he does not know what to say or, when asked a question, appears not to hear, drops his pencil or starts coughing. This boy may be showing signs of avoidance behaviour and withdrawal from the discomfort of stammering. In a class full of children, it is easy for this child to be passed over. When he withdraws from speech, you may move on to someone else, leaving the stammering child satisfied that he has escaped from exposing his speech problem, but frustrated that he has not answered a question to which he knew the answer.

These are only three examples of how different children might handle the situation. The way the child handles the episode of stammering is one indication of how he feels about the situation.

If there is an immediate crisis, it is often difficult to make the right long-term decision. I am reminded of a recent discussion with a group of nursery nurses. One of them broached the subject of 4-year-old Jonathan who invariably rushed up to her and hopped about threateningly from leg to leg while saying, 'Please may I go to the t——.' At this stage his speech would become quite blocked, his expression agonised and the nursery nurse felt the only thing to do was to say, 'Off you go to the toilet.' However, she also felt this might not be the ideal approach and so the matter was discussed. I asked whether she thought Jonathan was likely to have an accident on the floor. She doubted this. I then asked what she thought might be the long-term consequences of saying this word for him on each occasion? The pros and cons and various alternatives were aired and, as a group, we came to the conclusion that the next time Jonathan came rushing up the nursery nurse should wait calmly and patiently. True, Jonathan might have an accident either because he had waited too long and expected that he would be helped on his way, or because he would be utterly surprised by this change in reaction. In the long term, however, it was considered that Jonathan would attempt to say 'toilet' and not learn to use speech blockages to force others to speak for him or to opt out of speech.

Teachers may find the following suggestions helpful.

- Do not interfere directly with the child's speech by asking him to speak more slowly, take a deep breath, relax, and so on.
- Do keep your own speech calm and slow so that there is no challenge or threat of hurry.
- Take the focus off speech when there is difficulty. Let the

child finish what he is saying and then divert his attention to an activity other than speech at which he can succeed.

- Accept episodes of stammering as just 'one of those things'. This will help the stammering child and also set an example to other children.
- Do not exclude the child from speaking activities, but arrange matters according to his needs.
- Help the child to build his self-confidence by not over-emphasising speech and by finding positive aspects that can be praised.

Certain activities at school often pose special problems:

ANSWERING THE REGISTER

Recently a primary school teacher discussed a small boy whose surname began with an A, which placed him second on the register. This boy almost invariably stammered when answering the register and his teacher wondered whether to place him at the end of the roll-call so that he could hear a model of fluent answers before speaking himself. It is unlikely that this solution would prove helpful because, if left until the end, the boy might build fear and tension while waiting his turn. A different approach was suggested by another teacher.

She organised activities to take place at tables each morning and the children knew at which table to start the day. On calling the register each child would move to his allocated table, answering the register at some stage during this procedure. You might have thought of handling this situation differently, but the important aspects considered by the second teacher were:

- Putting emphasis on something other than speech.
- Allowing the child with a stammer to remain a part of the class activity.
- Minimising occasions when the class's attention is focused on the child struggling to say a word.

LEARNING TO READ

Some children actually start to stammer at the time of learning to read. This may be due to such things as difficulty with the early stages of reading, feelings of stress, general anxiety about school and so on. It is often a temporary phase, but stammering does occasionally persist. It is important to assess the real difficulty: is the child starting to stammer because he has a basic reading problem, or is the beginning of a stammer the real problem, and the child's reading adequate? There are times when a child does not receive help with a reading difficulty because it is thought that his reading is hampered by the stammer; there are other times when a child does not receive help with his stammer as it is assumed that his difficulty is with reading. A discussion between you and a speech therapist will enable a clear assessment to be made.

It will help the stammering child in the initial stages if there is an opportunity for the children to read individually to you.

The ideal is then to widen the situation with one other child. The stammering child is able to gain confidence with just one or two listeners while also gaining experience and competence in reading skills. If the child is showing some fluency while reading as well as gaining competence, he will more readily be able to read in front of others.

SPEAKING OR READING ALOUD IN CLASS

It is impossible to generalise about the management of these situations as so many variables have to be considered. However, in oral work, the following situations usually reduce stammering.

- When speaking or reading in unison.
- When speaking or reading with just one listener or within a small group.
- When speech is not the sole factor but is associated with some other activity.
- Speaking when there is no time pressure to complete the utterance quickly.
- Speaking on days when there is considerable fluency rather than days when fluency is at a minimum.

With young children and those relatively unconcerned by their stammer, much will depend on your management. With the older child, the child showing signs of real anxiety and the child who is well aware that he stammers, it is advisable to speak with the child alone so that his wishes may be considered. During such a talk, it is valuable to listen to the child, find out how he views his stammer and emphasise that you would like to help him to participate fully in class activities. The help that you could offer might be along such lines as discovering whether the child would prefer to speak near the start of an activity or not; whether he would like to have prior knowledge of the activity where possible so that he can prepare the work rather than speak impromptu; whether he would like to put up his hand when he wishes to make a contribution; and so on. You might also ask him whether, if the occasion arises, he would like the subject of stammering discussed in the classroom so that other children can gain information and understanding. Allowing the child some choice and listening to his viewpoint may alleviate a great deal of anxiety. The main purpose of such a talk is to let the child know that you are prepared to listen to him, are aware of his speaking difficulty, not particularly anxious about his stammer, and willing to help. If he is receiving therapy, it is important to find out whether he is working on a particular speech technique so that he may have your co-operation in using it in class. Unless you are certain that the child knows that he stammers and understands the meaning of the word, it is preferable not to use the term at first. It is better to use such phrases as 'Are you having some trouble with your speech?' or 'Do you sometimes get stuck when trying to say a word?' The child's answers can themselves be revealing.

Sometimes a child is quite unwilling to co-operate in such a discussion. It may be that the apparently uncooperative child is unconcerned by his stammer and so truly does not understand the purpose of the talk; at the other extreme, it may be that the child is unsure when talking to a teacher and so unwilling to expose himself, especially if he is anxious to hide his stammer.

TEASING

Although this can be minimised by your own example of acceptance, some teasing and giggling may still occur. Many children are teased at some stage at school. It is possible that certain children who stammer are highly sensitive to teasing because they do not know why they stammer or how to stop, and so the situation seems hopeless. An understanding teacher can be of great help. Many teachers do talk to the child and reassure him that he is doing well in many areas and so need not worry so much about the specific area of speech. The emphasis is on positive confidence building. If laughter occurs in class, it can be handled in the same way as when this happens if a child fails at geography, gets a sum wrong or cannot think of an example of a verb. If Johnny is asked to point to Paris on a wall map and he places Paris firmly in the middle of Southern India, laughter may ensue. What do you do then? You could do the same if there is laughter when a boy stammers. You probably take the former situation fairly casually, make some remark to quieten the class, reassure Johnny, and carry on. Treating stammering as just another aspect of behaviour rather than something special and dealing with it in the same fairly casual way is of infinite help to the stammerer and a useful lesson in tolerance for the other children. Providing the boy agrees and is well aware of his stammer, you might discuss the subject within the class. A lot of teasing stems from ignorance and explanations often help. I remember a 7-year-old who came home from school and described a great new game that was played in the playground. A whole lot of boys would chase another boy who had a piece of string hanging from his ear. Whenever anyone managed to pull this string out of his ear, the boy burst into tears. I explained about hearing loss and deafness and hearing-aids. I asked Anthony to put his hands over his ears and experience what it is like not to be able to hear properly. It was a revelation to him. He never attempted to pull at that hearing-aid again.

PTA MEETINGS

Many PTAs set aside certain meetings for discussion of child-related topics. Your local speech therapist may be willing to open a session on speech difficulties in general or stammering specifically. Although only 1–2 per cent of the population is thought to stammer, the seriousness of this condition for some people in adult life is often not understood. There are many men who believe that their social, economic and personal life is handicapped and constrained because of their stammer. They believe that they cannot express their personality adequately in relationships, cannot compete at work, cannot fulfil their potential. These men may have severe or mild stammers, but they *feel* disadvantaged. If a good understanding of stammering could be brought to teachers and parents, the development of damaging elements of the disorder could often be arrested. If there is no speech therapist available, contact the Association for Stammerers, who may be able to provide a guest speaker or some filmed material.

Perhaps the stammering child in your class would like to become a teacher, a mechanic, an actor or a draughtsman. If he has the ability, he can achieve his goal with or without a stammer but if, with your help, he can leave school without a chip on his shoulder about his speech then his path will be so much easier.

Chapter 8

The Special Problems of Teenagers

The teenage years are a time of change. Physically, emotionally, intellectually and socially the teenager is growing, developing and changing, but he rarely matures at the same rate in all areas and can be, for instance physically awkward whilst intellectually able, or physically capable whilst socially clumsy. Teenagers can appear overconfident and aggressively sure of themselves and yet, underneath it all, are often insecure and lacking in confidence. Many begin to worry desperately about their weight, height or hairstyle – sometimes to the exclusion of everything else. I am reminded of a 14-year-old with a hairstyle resembling a bird's nest because he had a mass of tight curls more like a guardsman's bearskin than hair. He was offered £10 by a misguided aunt to have his hair cut but, although this was then a large sum of money, he categorically refused the offer. He had reached a stage when he rejected adult interference with his personal tastes and decisions.

During this adolescent period, the young person often becomes oversensitive and self-conscious and has a great need to find praise and approval from those around him. He also becomes more objective, more able to stand outside himself, to make judgements and ask questions: 'What sort of person do I want to be? What do I like or dislike about myself and others? What do I want to do when I leave school? What sort of world am I living in?' He can be critical of adults in general, of his parents, of society and of the world we live in.

This questioning of himself and others can cause him to concentrate on his stammer at this time. Stammering usually starts in early childhood, but many children remain unconcerned by their speech difficulty until they reach adolescence. A teenage boy can gradually come to realise not only that he stammers, but the implications of this stammer on the social, emotional and economic sides of his life. Boys of 9 and 10 years rarely think along these lines but many teenagers do.

The changes that occur can be hard to handle and some parents find this an uncomfortable and difficult time. Their little boy who was polite, accepting and pleasant only a few months ago now seems to be forever arguing, challenging and brooding.

The needs of the teenager who stammers are the same as those of other teenagers and many excellent books have been written to give information and help to young people and adults. A recent, highly readable book on this subject is *Living with Teenagers – A Guide for the Perplexed* by Tom Crabtree (Futura Publications, 1980). The additional difficulties experienced by a teenager who stammers are obviously related to the greater need for communication as the child approaches manhood and to his own evaluation of that need.

The teenage stammerer may be in one of several situations.

The boy has been anxious about his stammer for some time and is receiving speech therapy

This teenager will have faced his stammer and is getting help and support with problems he may encounter.

The boy has been concerned about his stammer for some time, has been able to talk about this at home and school, but has received no therapy

It would be advisable to seek professional help.

The stammer is gradually improving and neither the teenager nor his family feels there is cause for concern

Then everything is going well and it is likely that this improvement will continue.

Although aware of his stammer for some time, the teenager has previously been unconcerned. There have been occasional references to stammering at home and at school, but it has not been an important issue and therapy has been thought unnecessary. The boy has now become worried about his speech and his stammer is worse. The changes in speech and attitude are difficult to handle

Help and advice should be sought from a speech therapist.

The stammer has not been discussed in the past because it was thought inadvisable to broach the subject. However, the stammer is well

established and the teenager seems tense and anxious when speaking.
There has been no previous therapy

It may be difficult to break down the wall of silence that has been created around the speech problem. A therapist's advice should be obtained so that stammering can be discussed and the boy receive help with his speech.

Speech therapy is usually extremely helpful for young people of this age. Sessions may be arranged individually on a once- or twice-weekly basis or in groups more intensively. Much will depend on the needs of each individual and on the speech therapy services available. The therapeutic techniques for teenagers are much the same as those for adults and will be described in Chapter 11. These techniques will be employed whether the therapy is on an individual or group basis. Groups may be organised to meet for one or more weeks during school holidays so that those who do not live in the immediate vicinity are able to join. Although work is generally centred on gaining fluency, considerable attention is also paid to discussion of both stammering and general topics of interest to teenagers – relationships, clothes, money, school, job prospects, the opposite sex, and so on. There will inevitably be a larger number of boys, but these groups also include girls who stammer. The young people can share their problems and realise that no one group member has difficulties that are totally unique. Although the therapist is there to lead, teach, guide and advise, considerable benefits are gained from the sharing which occurs between group members. Opportunities are usually given to develop the social skills of communication so that experience is acquired in using the telephone, talking to a headmaster, buying items in a shop, and so on. Most of these courses are run under the auspices of the National Health Service and are either free or entail a very small charge. It is often possible to obtain an allowance for fares and food costs so that no boy should be denied the opportunity of joining because his parents fear the financial outlay. It is always advisable to make inquiries about the services available in your area as regards both group and individual therapy. Contact your local speech therapist, your own doctor or, if experiencing difficulty, one of the addresses on page 118.

If it is impossible to obtain any therapeutic assistance, parents and teachers should be aware of the factors involved in order to help the child to help himself. Some of these factors are:

● Since most adults in his environment have known of the child's stammer for some time, it may be difficult to appreciate that he himself may only now begin to worry about how his speech may affect his everyday life. This can be disturbing to him, increase stammering and cause other changes – withdrawing from speech, talking too much, or feeling depressed or tense.

- The boy's feelings and attitude cannot be judged by the frequency and severity of his stammer. A boy who apparently has only an occasional, mild disruption in speech may be just as worried as one who has frequent, severe speech blockages.

- A great need of most teenagers is to find someone who can and will listen. If parents and teachers are available and able to listen rather than prejudge and offer solutions, this in itself will help the boy to clarify his anxieties and get the subject into proportion.

- A teenager likes to feel that he is understood as an individual, is given sufficient freedom to find out about life for himself and make his own decisions. If just told what to do, he may become hostile or withdrawn.

- Too many probing questions about his speech may not be useful. The teenager needs privacy and a chance to work things out for himself. Listening and understanding his point of view and then offering appropriate information and guidance will be of the greatest help.

If you are meeting problems with your teenager, then you are definitely not alone. A difficulty frequently encountered is that many families find it necessary to contain their problems and to present a picture of perfect harmony and bliss in front of others. Some parents actually close their eyes to problems in the vague hope that, if not acknowledged, they will somehow go away. Some years ago I was talking to a friend about our teenage children. She mentioned one of her boys who had started experimenting with drugs and talked about how guilty, ashamed and isolated she and her husband felt. After chatting for some considerable time, she said, 'You're the first friend I've been able to talk to because you are the only one who admits to having children who are not perfect. Everyone else always describes their perfect children, perfect relationships and perfect homes so that I just feel totally inadequate.' If you find yourself similarly isolated with regard to your son's stammer, speech therapists will offer support and information to parents as well as to teenagers.

The teenage years are a period of oscillation between childhood and adulthood with the resultant feelings of confusion and insecurity. This is a time when Johnny no longer sees himself as

Mr and Mrs Smith's little boy, but as John Smith – individual and unique. Although he may often speak and behave in such a way as to make it quite clear that his parents are old-fashioned, misguided, materialistic and rigid, he will still be in great need of their help and support. A teenager has many needs, but it is important that he understands that parents also have rights, including the right to enforce some of the rules by which they choose to live.

It has been said that it is what they *don't* know that hurts children. Worrying, wondering and guessing about the unknown can be far more harmful than clear discussion and information.

For this reason, here are some questions and comments often put by teenagers together with a basis for possible answers.

Why do I stammer?

A teenager can become almost obsessed with this question and this may be because he thinks that if a cause is found a cure cannot be far behind. In fact, it is highly unlikely that anyone will be able to pinpoint a single cause for a particular stammer. It is known that there is a tendency towards stammering in certain families; that there is a link between stammering and a slow learning of speech and language; that some parents become over-anxious about disfluency in early childhood, and so on. Even if it were possible to find the exact cause, it is unlikely that it would be of particular help. The child is now approaching manhood. The factors involved in the early stages of stammering may no longer be relevant and, at all events, will have changed considerably. Do not waste endless hours searching and worrying about the early beginnings. Look at the problem as it is now, today, and that will be a far better start to finding help or using the help you are already receiving.

Why do people assume that I'm stupid or incapable when I stammer?

This question often has an underlying but unspoken query about relationships with girls. It is important to be honest rather than deny this issue. There are some people who do look down on those who stammer just as they look down on anyone who has a difficulty or is in some way different from their accepted version of 'normal'. These people feel obliged to find something in others to criticise, pity or deprecate. Ask the teenager to describe a critical person that he knows and then to consider why that person needs to belittle others. Through discussion, the conclusion often reached is that this sort of individual is himself insecure and uncertain and needs to make others feel small in order to make himself feel big.

Sometimes criticism and snide remarks are due to ignorance about the subject so that the person sniping at a stammerer may be totally unaware of the distress being caused.

Since teenagers often overreact, it is helpful to establish exactly how many people, within the boy's own experience, have ever implied that he is stupid, inadequate or funny because he stammers. When pinpointed, it is often very few indeed. With this aspect in proportion, it is then possible to consider two points:

- The majority of people think of others as a whole human being and not just in terms of the stammer. It is unlikely that we make friends with someone solely because he has red hair, fluent speech, rich parents, and so on. Friends are made when people like a lot of things about each other – not just one thing.
- People tend to accept you as you present yourself. If you can take the stammer fairly lightly, others will be inclined to take the same view. If you are depressed and obsessed by your stammer, others may take their cue from you.

Will I grow out of my stammer?

Anything is possible. However, it is much more sensible to seek professional help so that definite steps can be taken to alleviate or cure this difficulty.

I had some speech therapy when I was 8 years old. It didn't help me then, why should it help now?

- Speech therapy may have helped at the age of 8 years. No one can tell whether the stammer would now be worse had there been no previous therapy.
- A lot of changes have taken place since you were 8 years old. You have changed, your stammer has changed, your attitude has changed and, possibly, the speech therapist has changed. Arguably, the most important change is that, at 8 years, some children are taken to see a speech therapist and may have little interest in their speech or in the therapy. Therefore the child has little motivation to work with the therapist. A teenager is capable of making his own decisions and, if he

decides to attend therapy, is able to co-operate fully with the therapist and the treatment plan.

I sometimes get very depressed and feel my life will be ruined by my stammer

Teenagers often get depressed and also suffer from mood swings – sometimes feeling very happy and then very depressed. The important point is that you do not sit around feeling more and more depressed, but try to do something. Write to the Association for Stammerers, find out about speech therapy, read a self-help book. The sooner you start to do something positive, the quicker you will begin to rid yourself of these unpleasant feelings.

The stammer stops me doing my best at school, especially in oral exams

Many teenagers feel that they are disadvantaged in some way. They are too fat or too thin, too big or too small, are growing too much hair or too little. They also feel that these characteristics are holding them back. Make sure that you are putting sufficient effort into your school work and not using the stammer as an excuse for not achieving higher results. Try to talk openly and honestly with a teacher so that something can be sorted out – especially regarding oral exams. Examiners can be told about your stammer in advance or you can tell them at the start of the exam so that you will not be hurried with your answers. Try to be well prepared so that you are confident about your knowledge of the subject. Finally, think before you speak, get your answer clear in your mind and then talk slowly without rush or panic. You should be all right.

I don't talk to anyone about my stammer. My parents won't listen, my teachers are too busy and my friends don't understand

Are you sure? Are you certain that neither of your parents will listen? Perhaps your mother or father might do so if you chose the right time. It is hard but, as you become older, some of the responsibility for the relationship with parents will depend on you and no longer solely on them. It would make a lot of difference to you and your parents if the subject of stammering could be brought into the open. Don't give up too quickly. See if you cannot find a way. The same applies to teachers. Are they *all* too busy? Is there one teacher to whom you could talk? Look at all the possibilities. If you could talk with one parent or one teacher, then that person could help you discuss the subject with someone else – a teacher might talk to your parents; a parent might talk with teachers. As for your friends, how much do you try to understand their troubles? If you can appreciate that they may feel just as badly about being fat, short of money or lonely as you do about stammering, this could develop into a two-way process. You listen to their worries and try to understand and they then listen and learn to understand about your stammer.

Will my stammer stop me getting a job?

Questions about job prospects have always been important to teenagers. At the present time with world-wide recession and high unemployment in the United Kingdom, these questions are even more central. The particular question asked here has two basic features:

Will I get a job at all in this time of high unemployment? There is no easy answer. Much will depend on the teenager's qualifications, personality, the geographical area in which he lives and the political climate at the time he is job-hunting.

Will I get a job with my stammer? Again, there is no easy answer. The fact is that the majority of adult stammerers are employed in all possible fields – as teachers, decorators, civil servants, solicitors, computer operators, and so on. There are many factors involved when answering this question. How severe is the stammer? How frequent is the stammer? How anxious is the boy about his stammer? Does he view it as a handicap or is it fairly unimportant to him? Is he receiving any help with his speech? These questions, together with those specially geared to job prospects, will determine any individual's work potential. However, the boy is still in his teens and presumably at school so help at this stage can affect his long-term prospects and this is a further reason why therapy is advisable.

This chapter has focused on the 'special problems' of teenagers and therefore little has been said about the 'special advantages' of teenagers. Although adults associated with this age-group can become exasperated, defensive and anxious, they also find challenge and reward. Teenagers are searching, discovering and experimenting – there is excitement in these years and the rewards of seeing the young person developing into a thinking, caring and achieving young man are indeed high.

Chapter 9

For Adults – Getting to Know Your Stammer

This chapter explains the individual nature of stammering so that the relevance of various therapeutic approaches can be better understood. It is intended to help adults, some teenagers — particularly those in the older age groups – and those trying to help themselves in the absence of speech therapy.

By this stage, you will have stammered for some years and, although aware of this, you may have spent so much time hiding and avoiding your stammer that you have not been in touch with the details of your speech difficulty. Alternatively, your stammer may be frequent and severe so that your energies have been channelled into trying to communicate; often you become quite exhausted with the effort. In the event, few people ever look closely at what they actually do when stammering.

You may believe that it is not what you do but what happens to you that constitutes the difficulty. Consider for a moment the statement that 'stammering is what you do in order to stop stammering'. For adults and confirmed stammerers there is much truth in it. Take for example a man who wants to say, 'Can you tell me the way to the nearest underground station?' Before asking the question, the man considers that he will be unable to get started because he has difficulty with the 'c' of 'can'. He decides to change the question to 'Would you tell me the way to the nearest underground station?' Having stopped someone in the street and started speaking, he suddenly becomes aware that he will be unable to say 'station'. He is committed. The listener is waiting, the speaker has got as far as 'Would you tell me the way . . . .'. He has no time to think things through and so makes a somewhat panicky decision to change the sentence around in order to avoid the feared word. He ends up saying, 'Would you tell me the way to the nearest place to get an underground?' Much of what this man did was in order to stop himself stammering. He succeeded by means of altering and avoiding the feared words. Take the same man when, later in the day, he is asked:

'What is your name?' The name is John Smith and he invariably stammers on the 'j' of 'John'. He has tried many ways of stopping himself stammering on this sound, but has rarely succeeded. He tries to rush through the feared word by dint of saying: 'Well you see actually my name is J–J–John Smith.' The 'j' of 'John' is forced out in a burst of speed and with considerable tension. On this occasion he still stammered. Nevertheless, much of what he did was in order to stop himself stammering – he used unnecessary words, increased the speed of speech and forced out the word 'John' with extra pressure and tension.

Adult stammerers often have strong feelings about their speech, but find looking closely at what they actually do distressing. So life goes on with fear, embarrassment and anxiety and without any precise examination of the situation.

It is difficult to rid oneself of any form of behaviour or to change it unless the nature of that behaviour is clear. For this reason, many types of therapy and self-therapy involve some work on defining the patterns of an individual's stammer. When working without a therapist, in order to help with this process it is useful to have a mirror and a tape recorder. When by yourself, it may be impossible to stammer so try to think yourself into a situation in which you recently had trouble and imitate the stammer that occurred. Watch what you do in the mirror and listen to what you can hear on tape. It will take time but, gradually, you will begin to note certain features. The first steps may be painful and unpleasant because you will become more aware of what you are doing and get closer to your difficulty than you have before. Once the initial steps are taken, you will know that you are doing something positive on the path to facing and alleviating your problem.

The following questionnaire is designed as an aid in defining various common features. (Not all features will apply to each stammerer.)

1   What are you doing?

(a) *Blocking*   The sound or word gets 'stuck'. You cannot go on speaking and probably have to 'push' the word out. If this applies, do you:

   (i)   block and no sound comes out?
   (ii) block and make a sound or noise of some sort?
   (iii) are there any particular sounds on which you usually block? If so, what are they?

(b) *Repeating*   Saying the same sound or group of sounds over and over again (m–m–m–m–mother or bu–bu–butter). If so, do you repeat:

(i)   sounds (b–b–b–butter)?
(ii) syllables (bu–bu–bu–butter)?
(iii) both the above?

(c) *Prolonging* Holding on to a sound (fffffffather or Sssssssaturday). If so, which sounds:

m, s, sh, z, r, l or others?

2   How often do you stammer?

(i)   Very often – once every two or three words or every sentence.
(ii) Quite often – once every few minutes.
(iii) Not very often – a few times during the day.
(iv) Rarely – a few times during one week.
(v)   Very rarely – on the odd sounds in a particular situation: perhaps on the telephone, at a meeting or only with certain people.
(vi) Hardly at all – sometimes not for weeks and then quite mildly.
(vii) In some other way.

3   How bad is it?

(i)   You get completely 'stuck', lose control over your speech and cannot go on.
(ii) You manage to attempt the sound or make some kind of noise, but take quite a time to say the word.
(iii) You repeat a sound or word several times, but go on with what you want to say.
(iv) You have mild hesitations, but carry on with what you want to say quite easily.
(v)   You find your stammer hardly interrupts the flow of speech.

4   How tense do you feel?

(i)   Very tense.
(ii) Fairly tense.
(iii) Not very tense.
(iv) Not tense.
(v)   Sometimes tense and sometimes relaxed.
(vi) Other than the above.

The answers to the above questions will give you some idea of certain features of your particular stammer. You may find that you have quite severe blocks, which considerably interrupt what you want to say, but which happen fairly infrequently. Or you may find that the interruptions are so severe and frequent that you lose track of what you want to say. Perhaps you cannot be certain because some days the stammer is very frequent and severe and other times you are very fluent. You may discover that it is difficult to answer the questions as you do all these things some of the time because everything depends on the specific situation or particular person with whom you find yourself.

The answers to these questions give some indication of the severity of your difficulty. Speech therapists would assess this by considering the kind of stammer, the frequency, the duration and the amount of tension. It is important to appreciate that, for therapists and clients alike, this is only one part of an assessment and other factors will be discussed in the next chapter.

A general guide against which to check your answers is given opposite.

FLUENCY

Just as important as the stammer is that other aspect of speech – *fluency*. How fluent are you? When are you fluent? In what way are you fluent. How much of the time are you fluent? It is worth thinking about this. Stammering is often such a nuisance and so emotive that it is natural to think solely about the stammer and not the periods of fluent speech. It is like that in life when for weeks nothing particularly startling may happen. During the day you go to school or to work; in the evening you go home, to the pub or the pictures, and it is all routine and ordinary. If someone says 'What sort of week have you had?' you may answer 'Quite ordinary – just the usual.' But if during that week you go to the pub or a disco and someone takes a punch at you, you will register this, even though you were not hurt. That punch interrupted the usual routine of life in a sudden and possibly unpleasant manner. The same applies to stammering – fluency is the routine flow of speech which, whether we stammer or not, is taken for granted. The stammer is the punch – painful or not, severe or not, it interrupts the normal progress of speech and so is registered. Because fluency is mostly taken for granted, you may find it difficult to consider this feature of your speech. It is useful to have a notebook and keep it by you for a few days so that notes can be made on how fluent you are during the day, with whom and in what situations.

	Very Mild	Mild	Mild to Moderate	Moderate	Moderate to Severe	Severe	Very Severe
The amount of stammering	Less than 1% of words	1–2% of words	2–5% of words	5–8% of words	8–12% of words	12–25% of words	More than 25% of words
The duration of the stammer	Less than 1 second	Approx. 1 second	Mostly 1 second	Approx. 1 second	Approx. 2 seconds	Average 3–4 seconds	Average more than 4 seconds
The type of stammer	Repetitions	Repetitions	Mostly repetitions, some blocks/prolongations	Mostly repetitions but some blocks/prolongations	Blocks – perhaps repetitions/prolongations	Blocks – perhaps repetitions/prolongations	Blocks – with or without repetitions/prolongations
Tension	Very little	Very little	Some, but not distracting	Some, occasionally distracting	Frequent	Conspicuous	Severe

(The above scale is condensed from Johnson, W., Darley, F. L., and Spriesterbach, D. C., *Diagnostic Methods in Speech Pathology* (1963).)

5   How much fluency?

(i)   Hardly any – stammering on most words most of the time.
(ii)   Not very much – fluent with certain people at certain times only.
(iii) Quite a lot – speaking fluently for quite long periods of time.
(iv)   A lot – short episodes of stammering but fluent most of the time.
(v)   Most of the speech is fluent.
(vi)   Other than the above.

6   What sort of fluency?

(i)   When fluent, speech feels natural and normal.
(ii)   Even when fluent, feeling only one step away from stammering.
(iii) When fluent, feeling it is different from other people's fluency.
(iv)   Other than the above.

7   What percentage of fluency?

(i)   90 per cent.
(ii)   75 per cent.
(iii) 50 per cent.
(iv)   35 per cent.
(v)   Less than 35 per cent.

You may feel quite cheerful after answering questions 5–7 as perhaps you have discovered that not only is there more fluency in your speech than you had thought but you feel like a normal speaker when fluent. In that case, you may have a mild stammer. Conversely, you may have found that there is little fluency and that the fluency never *feels* right. This could be associated with a more severe stammer. Or it may have become apparent that although there is a considerable amount of fluency you never feel safe from stammering even when fluent. Perhaps some clues to your difficulty will be found in the next chapter.

Are you beginning to feel that all this is totally irrelevant? After all, a stammer is a stammer. At the risk of labouring the point – no, a stammer is not just a stammer. Your stammer is different in some way, however slightly, from other people's stammers. It will help you to know your own stammer whether you are working with a therapist or on your own.

COMMUNICATION

How much does the stammer prevent you from communicating your thoughts to other people? Communication is what speech is all about. We think of something to say and put our thoughts into words in order to communicate these thoughts to others. An unwanted interruption in this process is a disadvantage.

8   How much does the stammer interfere with communication?

  (i)   Hardly at all – you generally say what you want to say when you want to say it.
 (ii)   A fair amount – you sometimes know what you want to say, but do not say it for fear of stammering.
(iii)   Quite a lot – you often know what you want to say, but do not say it for fear of stammering.
 (iv)   Most of the time – you think about your stammer most of the time and this stops you communicating spontaneously.
  (v)   All the time – you are never at ease when speaking.

Question 8 raises a fundamental issue. There are many annoying things about stammering. One of the most crucial is how much communication is impaired because of the stammer. It would seem obvious that the more severe and frequent the occurrence, the more communication is impaired. It is not always so simple. Some people with mild speech problems still find communication difficult. Others with apparently more severe speech problems find it easier to communicate.

Check your answers:

(i) or (ii)   – a good ability to communicate
(iii)   – communication brings considerable difficulty
(iv) or (v) – severe communication difficulty

The answers to questions 1–8 will give you insight into certain areas – what you do when you stammer, the fluency in your speech and your overall communicative ability. The next chapter will look at different but equally important issues.

Chapter 10

More About Your Stammer

EMOTIONAL ASPECTS

As stammering fully develops in teenage and adulthood, feelings and emotions become involved and the problem is no longer merely one of producing a smooth flow of words. To understand the nature of stammering in general and your own difficulty in particular, and to obtain help or help yourself, you will need to examine closely the feelings you experience.

Some stammerers assume that all others feel exactly as they do – embarrassed, stupid, guilty, ashamed or whatever. This is not so. Some feel cross, some embarrassed, while others are not unduly concerned about their speech. Everyone is unique – an individual.

Therapists examine the *overt* and *covert* factors in stammering. The overt factors are the external and outward ones – speech and the general signs of difficulty which can be seen and heard by the listener and felt by the speaker. These factors are investigated in questions 1–8 in Chapter 9. The covert factors are the internal or inner difficulties which cannot be seen or heard by the listener and may or may not be known to the speaker.

Perhaps these terms can be clarified by an analogy formulated by Dr Joseph Sheehan, who likened stammering to an iceberg. Part of an iceberg can be clearly seen above the surface of the water, but another and sometimes more dangerous part is hidden below the surface of the water. Although hidden beneath the surface, this is an integral part of the whole iceberg. Stammering can be viewed in the same way. Like an iceberg, there is the outward part that can be seen and heard and the hidden portion that is submerged below the surface.

Here are some examples of such icebergs:

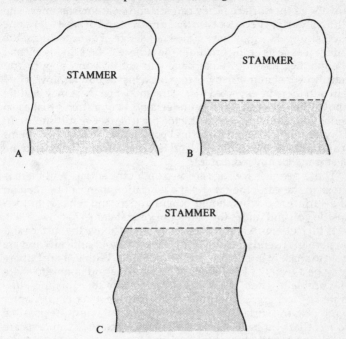

Everything above the line is the overt, visible and audible part of stammering. Everything below that line is covert, hidden, internal and not seen or heard by other people.

Iceberg A illustrates the situation often found in small children and some older ones. Theirs is mainly a speech problem. Children have not accumulated much experience of disfluency and often attach little importance to it, so that they are not necessarily concerned or worried. The speech problem is mostly of a simple nature because it is above the surface.

Iceberg B illustrates the situation for an older child, teenager or adult. There is a considerable amount of stammering and, beneath the surface, some anxiety such as fear of stammering, anticipation of trouble, and the habit of stammering on certain sounds and in certain situations, etc.

Then there is iceberg C, which is largely submerged. This type of iceberg causes distress to seafarers and it is also a source of distress to the stammerer. In this situation there is relatively little outward stammering, but considerable fear and anxiety under the surface.

The rest of the world can see and hear the outward features that are above the surface. They can see and hear the stammer. The difficulty arises because even those nearest and dearest – let alone total strangers – may have little knowledge of your feelings, the internal aspects going on under the surface. Often clients tell me: 'People keep saying, what have you got to worry about? You hardly ever stammer; you're making a fuss about nothing.' How can outsiders be expected to understand when there may be little above the surface? Do you understand why a friend makes so much fuss about his ears being too big (they seem quite normal); why a friend constantly worries because she is too fat (she seems just right); or why another friend feels he is not well educated (he seems most knowledgeable)?

These people's feelings are also under the surface and there is more to the ears, the fat and the education than can be seen on the surface. So why should others understand what is hidden inside you and under the surface of your stammer?

With icebergs A and B there is quite a lot above the surface and so perhaps friends and relatives talk about your difficulty and are able to share at least some of your problems. With iceberg C there may be a feeling of isolation, of being alone and unable to share the problem. There are many stammerers in the situation illustrated by iceberg C. The guide to stammering severity in Chapter 9 refers to the surface or overt symptoms, but it is quite possible to *feel* that you have a severe stammer when the symptoms are mostly covert and below the surface.

Here are some questions which may help you to map out your own iceberg:

9   How much avoidance do you use?

Do you use the following:

(i)   Certain sounds or words. For example, do you say 'small' instead of 'little' or 'town' when you wish to say 'city'?

(ii)   Certain subjects. For example, when asked by a stranger what sort of holiday you have had, do you answer 'quite good' when you wished to say that you 'had a marvellous time in Malta'?

(iii)   Certain situations. For example, do you go to the supermarket instead of a shop where you have to ask for your goods? Do you hand over the exact fare instead of asking for your destination?

(iv)   Certain people. For example, do you avoid your headmaster, your boss, or others?

If so, do you do this:

(a) Rarely – only on very few occasions if at all?
(b) Quite a lot – several times each day?
(c) Frequently – almost every time when you feel you will stammer?

10 How much do you talk?

(i) As much as you want and when you want.
(ii) Quite a lot, but occasionally when wishing to speak you opt out and stay silent.
(iii) Not a lot – you tend not to speak unless you have to do so.
(iv) As little as possible – only when absolutely essential.

11 Do you use tricks to postpone or to help start speech?

(a) Do you use 'starters'? Do you insert 'm' or 'er' to get speech started, or use a favourite phrase ('you know'; 'well, you see'; 'actually')?

If so, which of the following?

(i) m
(ii) er
(iii) a particular word or phrase
(iv) some other device to get speech started

(b) Do you take 'a run' into words? If you find difficulty with a word, do you go back and take 'a run' at it (once upon a t—— once upon a t—— once upon a time)?

If so, do you do this:

(i) rarely?
(ii) quite often?
(iii) frequently?

(c) Do you use physical tricks to start speech, for example coughing, foot-tapping, pretending not to hear, etc.

If so, do you do this:

(i) rarely?
(ii) quite often?
(iii) frequently?

12 What do you feel when you stammer?

   (i)   Nothing very much.
  (ii)   Embarrassed.
 (iii)   Anxious.
 (iv)   Guilty.
   (v)   Angry.
 (vi)   Other than the above.

   If you have these feelings, are they:

   (i)   Mild – occur quite rarely and are not distressing.
  (ii)   Moderate – *either* occur rarely but are strong when they
         happen *or* occur frequently but are not strong feelings.
 (iii)   Severe – occur frequently and are strong feelings.

13 How did you buy or borrow this book?

   (i)   Asked the assistant for a book on stammering.
  (ii)   Looked on the shelves, but did not want to ask the
         assistant.
 (iii)   Looked on the shelves, but felt anxious about what the
         assistant or librarian might think.
 (iv)   Got a friend/relative to find it.
   (v)   Some other way.

Questions 9 and 10 are concerned with avoidance behaviour.
The more you avoid, particularly people and situations, the
greater your need to hide the fact that you stammer. This may be
because in answering Questions 12 and 13 you find that you feel
guilty or ashamed about stammering and cannot bear others to
know about it.

Question 10 is also related to the overall speech pattern.
Someone who talks very rarely may also stammer rarely solely
because he is speaking as little as possible. Another person may
talk a considerable amount and feel free to say what he wishes.
The amount of stammering may then apparently be greater
because there is much more speech. Therefore, it is important to
view the amount of stammering in relation to the amount of
talking.

Question 11 deals with some aspects of how you cope with
your stammer. If you go straight into the stammer without
withdrawing or recoiling from it, you are allowing your stammer
to remain above the surface. However, if you use any number of
postponing or starting devices, some of your stammer will be
hidden. Others may well not realise that you were going to
stammer because some trick made you sound fluent.

Tricks and devices are sometimes inevitable but, if these are used frequently, again there is a need to hide the stammer for reasons that may or may not have become apparent when answering Question 12.

From the information and questions in this and the previous chapter, you may like to fill in your own iceberg and see whether it is like iceberg A, B or C.

EXAMPLES

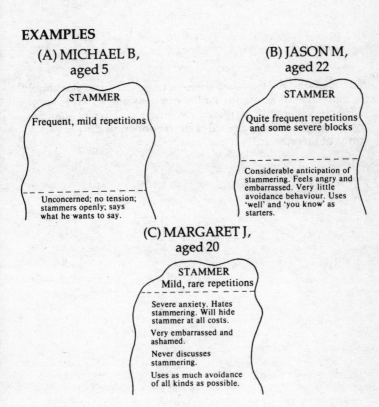

(A) MICHAEL B, aged 5

STAMMER

Frequent, mild repetitions

- - - - - - - - - - - - - - -

Unconcerned; no tension; stammers openly; says what he wants to say.

(B) JASON M, aged 22

STAMMER

Quite frequent repetitions and some severe blocks

- - - - - - - - - - - - - - -

Considerable anticipation of stammering. Feels angry and embarrassed. Very little avoidance behaviour. Uses 'well' and 'you know' as starters.

(C) MARGARET J, aged 20

STAMMER
Mild, rare repetitions
- - - - - - - - - - - - - - -

Severe anxiety. Hates stammering. Will hide stammer at all costs.

Very embarrassed and ashamed.

Never discusses stammering.

Uses as much avoidance of all kinds as possible.

CAN YOU FILL IN YOUR OWN ICEBERG?

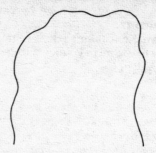

Now that you have worked through these chapters, you should be more able to assess the nature of your stammer. This knowledge, together with increased awareness of different stammering patterns, will help towards a clearer understanding of various forms of therapy.

Chapter 11

Theories and Therapies

This chapter describes and explains methods currently used by speech therapists and the rationale for their use, and gives information about the background as well as the practicalities of stammering therapy.

ISSUES IN STAMMERING THERAPY

When starting therapy, a client may be asked: 'What do you mean by a cure?' The most usual answers are of two kinds: 'I want to be totally fluent' or 'I can cope with some degree of stammering, but want to be able to speak without fear or worry'. This question and the answers underline the individual nature of the disorder. People differ in what they want from therapy and, although certain features predominate, stammering patterns differ too.

In 1939 the late Dr Wendell Johnson wrote: 'There is no such thing as *the* method for treating stuttering, and the fact that so many different methods are more or less successful is of more than incidental interest.' There is still no such thing as *the* method in the treatment of stammering. Sometimes there is an item in the newspaper describing yet another 'miracle' cure for stammering. The hopes of stammerers are raised on reading that Mr X or Mr Y was totally cured of his speech impediment by this particular method. Yet investigation usually shows that this 'miracle' cure had little long-lasting benefit or that it was beneficial only to Mr X and Mr Y. Stammering remains a mysterious disorder and, as such, lends itself to extravagant claims that someone somewhere has invented the quick, simple cure. In reality, there is little that is new in stammering therapy, but technology has improved and research by dedicated professionals in many fields has given a clearer understanding of why and how some methods are more effective than others.

AIMS OF THERAPY

When first thinking about therapy, most clients believe that its purpose is simple and obvious – to create fluency as quickly and efficiently as possible. Professional and non-professional workers alike have striven tirelessly with this aim in mind, using methods as diverse as the rhythmic timing of speech, the administration of electric shocks, the encouragement of relaxation, the use of drugs and speech drills, and so on. These methods have been used not for years but for centuries and are aimed at *establishing* fluency.

Only recently have speech therapists become aware that most stammerers can become fluent in a short time by the use of any number of therapeutic techniques, but that the *establishment* of fluency is only one step. Considerable attention is now focused on three stages – the *establishment*, *transfer* and *maintenance* of fluency. Establishment means teaching the stammerer to speak fluently within the clinic and with a therapist; transfer is the promotion of fluent speech in a variety of situations with a range of listeners; maintenance is the continued use of fluent speech for a long period of time after regular therapy has stopped.

Some disagreement appears to relate to *how* fluency should be established, but the differences are really about how fluency can be established so that it will be *maintained* throughout the person's life. This must be the issue. When a man says that he wants to become fluent or to be able to speak without fear, he is talking about the rest of his life and not about the next few days or months. He is talking about his life in his own world and not about a few hours, weeks or months spent in a clinic or centre.

Looking back at the icebergs and the questions considered in previous chapters, it will be apparent that stammering in adulthood is rarely a simple speech disorder as there are many different sorts of stammers – from mild to severe – and many different ways of feeling about a stammer. It is a simple matter to draw icebergs on paper, but the icebergs of stammerers are not formed with paper and pencil, nor do they float randomly in the waters of an arctic ocean. The stammer depicted in the form of an iceberg is an integral part of a person with that individual's background, personality, attitudes, achievements, hopes and fears.

Consider iceberg A with largely overt or outward stammering behaviour as contrasted with iceberg C with mainly covert or hidden features. There is a school of thought which believes that, regardless of the different features of these icebergs, the client says that he stammers and so the duty of a therapist is to help him eliminate the overt features which constitute the seen and heard aspects of his speech difficulty. Other therapists believe that if, as in icebergs B and C, a considerable part of the stammer is hidden and concerned with feelings and attitudes, then therapy must be designed to help the stammerer with those covert feelings and attitudes as well as with the overt stammering symptoms.

Dr Hugo Gregory gives a full account of current thinking on these conflicting opinions in his book *Controversies about Stuttering Therapy*. He differentiates what he calls the 'speak more fluently' and the 'stammer more fluently' approaches to therapy. The 'speak more fluently' group of therapies have as their fundamental reasoning: This is a man who stammers, he has come to see us in order to become a fluent speaker, therefore, we will use our knowledge and expertise to teach him to 'speak more fluently'. When he can speak more fluently, his fears may well diminish and his attitudes change.

The 'stammer more fluently' group of therapies have as their fundamental reasoning: This is a man who stammers, he has come to see us with the outward features of a stammer, but also with associated fears and attitudes which he has nurtured for many years. If we content ourselves with teaching him to 'speak more fluently' we will have tackled the surface symptoms but the fears beneath the surface may remain. The client may already be avoiding and hiding his stammer and if we only teach him a fluency technique we may add a further means to hide and avoid, whilst doing nothing to resolve the hidden or underlying features of his problem. Therefore our aim should be to help this man face and understand his stammer, and learn not to fear and hide it but to modify and weaken it gradually so that he can 'stammer more fluently'.

THE MAINTENANCE OF FLUENCY

The 'speak more fluently' school of thought concentrates on establishing fluency efficiently and quickly so that this fluency can be transferred and maintained in the client's own environment.

The 'stammer more fluently' school of thought does not aim at maintenance of *fluency*, but at maintaining a positive attitude to speech so that the avoidance of words and situations and the fear of speech are gradually eliminated. This change to a more positive attitude will enable the stammerer to use techniques designed to help him to approach rather than to avoid stammering and to lessen the struggle and tension of stammering when it occurs. In this way it is thought that there will be a gradual modification of the total stammering syndrome – the stammer and the feelings associated with stammering.

SUMMARY

Stammering therapy can now be seen in terms of a preference for one of the two major approaches – the 'speak more fluently' or the 'stammer more fluently'. However, more and more therapists are coming to believe that the advantages of both methods can be combined and that it is possible both to establish fluency and to help the stammerer to adopt a more positive attitude to his speech, with better results than if one approach or the other were used alone.

Fluency cannot be maintained easily by the adult stammerer and much work will be required both of him and his therapist in order to achieve it. But the continuing research of therapists, together with the co-operation of stammerers, is leading to a greater understanding of the problem, and the realisation that the two main approaches in the treatment of stammering can be used hand in hand promises a brighter outlook for the future.

THE STRUCTURE OF THERAPY

The two main approaches are taught in somewhat different ways. Therapy for the 'speak more fluently' methods is generally provided in highly organised and clearly defined stages. The progression to fluency is achieved in small, precise steps so that the client moves from one stage to the next always developing and extending his newly learned pattern of fluent speech. In the United States programmes are available for therapist and client to follow, and are structured to increase fluency in the most efficient and systematic way possible. In the United Kingdom certain therapists have attended courses in one of these – the Monterey Fluency Programme devised by Bruce Ryan and Barbara van Kirk. This programme works through three modes of speech – reading, monologue and conversation – and, when the client has established fluency at each level, he progresses to the transfer and maintenance programmes. Whether fluency techniques are taught within such a totally structured framework or not, the 'speak more fluently' therapy methods are based on working step by step so that the fluency learned is used first in easy and then in more difficult situations.

The 'stammer more fluently' approaches cannot be so precisely structured. There is more emphasis on discussion between client and therapist so that the client can provide information on his problem and practise the techniques he learns, while the therapist can use her skills to help the specific difficulties of the client both in modifying his stammering pattern and in decreasing his fears of speech. Procedures are not followed precisely as is done when a 'speak more fluently' programme is used. 'Stammer more fluently' therapists prefer to work on an individualised basis – even working within a group – so that known techniques can be adapted to the needs of clients.

PRACTICAL CONSIDERATIONS

Clients may be offered therapy on an individual basis or within a group of approximately 3–9 people. This is not necessarily an either-or situation as, in some instances, it is thought advisable to start treatment individually and then continue within a group, or to do some individual work at the same time as group therapy, or to begin with group therapy and then continue on an individual basis. There are obvious advantages and disadvantages to both group and individual work. The main advantages of individual therapy are that the client and therapist can get to know each other so that the treatment can be adapted to the requirements of the client, and that the client can feel relaxed and secure when working with just one other person. The advantages of group work are that group members come to realise that their problems are not unique and that others share their difficulties; a wider range of speech experiences can be provided in a group of people than on an individual basis; and members of a group can learn from each other as well as from the therapist.

Both individual and group treatment can be given on an intensive or non-intensive basis. Intensive work would involve anything from 3 sessions per week lasting from 30 minutes to several hours per day. Non-intensive treatment involves sessions of varying lengths of time on one day per week or fortnight. Not only are there advantages and disadvantages, but the nature of therapy must be considered. Some forms of treatment are more suited to intensive work, and other methods are more effective on a non-intensive schedule.

TREATMENT METHODS

'SPEAK MORE FLUENTLY' APPROACHES

TECHNIQUES ASSOCIATED WITH DELAYED AUDITORY FEEDBACK

When speaking, we hear the words we say at the time that they are spoken. With delayed auditory feedback (DAF), the speaker talks into a microphone, a machine records his speech and this is then fed back to him through earphones a fraction of a second after it would normally be heard. Under DAF the majority of stammerers become fluent, but their speech is not exactly like normal speech because the rate is slow and there is a marked prolongation of the sounds spoken. The slow, prolonged pattern produced is due to the speaker trying to keep in tune with the delayed feedback he is receiving.

This fluent pattern of speech can be created in many stammerers by using a DAF machine. Some therapists use such a machine to establish fluency and, as the delay is gradually reduced, the client is helped to increase the rate of speech and shorten the prolongations until normal-sounding speech is achieved. The client is then instructed to continue using this fluent speech pattern without the aid of a machine.

This method is effective for many stammerers, but only a few therapists have access to a DAF machine. It has been found feasible and successful to teach this type of slow/prolonged speech without the use of a machine. The following description of this technique gives some indication of what is involved.

SLOW/PROLONGED SPEECH

This is a fluency-shaping method commonly used in the United Kingdom and other parts of the world for helping stammerers to achieve control over their speech. It is based on the sort of speech produced under DAF conditions and alters certain characteristics that contribute to stammering. People stammer in many different ways, but some features predominate. Take for example one such feature, which is that a stammerer is often very urgent about speech. His speech may be generally fast, or there may be bursts of speed when he anticipates a stammer or just after a stammer has occurred. Many people who stammer *feel* urgent about their speech. One man described this by saying, 'I feel like an express train inside: I've got to keep going, keep going, keep going.'

The aim of slow/prolonged speech is that the client learns all or some of the following aspects simultaneously:

Slowing down the rate of speech Slowing down the rate of speech has been found to be a strong aid to reducing stammering. Speed is gradually increased as the technique becomes more firmly established.

Using adequate pausing   Most people who stammer dread silence in speech and tend to become extremely urgent to complete an utterance quickly whilst they are able to speak. Fear of interruption may also contribute to lack of pausing. Normal pausing is helpful in changing the urgent quality of stammered speech.

Making light contacts   'Contacts' refers to the touching of any two speech organs or 'articulators' in order to produce a particular sound (see illustration). To make a 'p' or 'b' sound, the lips have to touch; to make a 't' or 'd' sound, the tip of the tongue touches the hard palate just behind the upper teeth; for an 'f' or 'v' sound, the lower lip touches the upper teeth, etc. The object here is to help in the production of light, relaxed contacts and eliminate the tense, hard contacts which contribute to stammering.

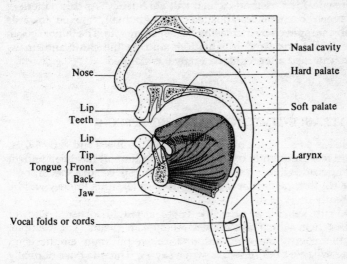

CONTACTS MADE BY THE SPEECH ORGANS IN THE PRODUCTION OF
SOME CONSONANTS

Air is breathed in through the nose and mouth, passes into the lungs and is then exhaled. In speech, as air is exhaled and passes through the larynx (at the level of the Adam's apple) where the vocal cords are situated, the air may activate the vocal cords so that they vibrate and voice is produced. The sounds of speech are then formed on the air stream, by changes in the position of the speech organs (illustrated). Consonant sounds are produced by contact between speech organs. Many of the sounds are illustrated in pairs as they are formed by similar contacts and only differ because one is voiced (the vocal cords vibrate) and the other is voiceless (no vibration), for example p, t and s are voiceless whilst their twins b, d and z are voiced. We rarely make sounds in isolation and the transition between sounds is so fast that this difference is not apparent during speech.

Achieving a smooth flow of speech   Although a smooth flow of words is characteristic of fluent speech, many stammerers seem to tackle each word separately so that their speech has a jerky quality. When smooth, flowing speech is produced, a more normal speaking pattern is established.

Prolonging speech sounds   The prolongation or elongation of some sounds, particularly the vowel sounds, makes it easier to pass smoothly from one sound to the next – an aspect of speech which is difficult for some stammerers.

As slow/prolonged speech is learnt – either in its entirety or in part – fluency and control of speech increase. Features in speech which contribute to stammering are replaced by more appropriate speaking methods which will aid fluency. As this pattern of speech becomes established, it is gradually moved towards normal speech by increasing the speaking rate. The fluent speech is then transferred to situations outside the clinic and finally maintained after regular therapy has stopped.

SYLLABLE-TIMED OR SYLLABIC SPEECH

This is a technique much favoured in the 1960s and early 1970s, but less frequently used at the present time. It has been known for decades that if a stammerer times his speech to a specific beat or rhythm he will become fluent, or at least his fluency will be greatly increased.

With syllabic speech, the client is taught to use a form of speech in which all syllables are spoken evenly. For example, when saying the word 'importance' we put more emphasis on the syllable underlined, or when saying 'Thursday' we normally emphasise the first syllable – 'Thursday'. In syllabic speech, all syllables are given the same emphasis and each is said in time to a regular rhythm. Some therapists use a metronome to help the client speak syllable by syllable in time to the beat. It is equally possible to acquire this technique without the use of a metronome.

The technique is taken in small steps so that the rate of speech is gradually increased, normal emphasis of syllables is brought back into speech, and more complex speech situations are introduced.

Although syllabic speech has proved successful for certain stammerers, many therapists now prefer to teach slow/prolonged

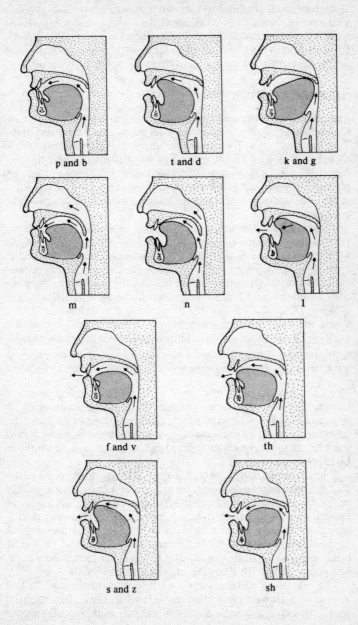

p and b

t and d

k and g

m

n

l

f and v

th

s and z

sh

speech because studies have shown that, whereas syllabic speech establishes fluency in a very short time, the transfer and maintenance is often unsatisfactory. The client must time his speech to a regular rhythm, and he often feels that this sounds abnormal and so does not readily speak in this way outside the clinic.

AIRFLOW TECHNIQUE

The airflow technique is clearly described in *Stuttering Solved* by Dr Martin Schwartz, and only a brief outline will be given here. This method is based on the assumption that stammering is due to various factors which cause the vocal cords to close tightly. According to Dr Schwartz, the stammerer's problem is that, in trying to release himself from this tightness or spasm in his vocal cords, he struggles and tenses and so stammering speech is produced.

The treatment, which again is taken in small, graded steps, begins when the client is asked to produce a long, audible sigh, which releases the tension in the vocal cords. He is then asked to sigh again and, when half-way through the sigh, to say a one-syllable word. When this is said fluently and easily, the number of one-syllable words is increased while the client is instructed to make the flow of air inaudible. Eventually it becomes possible to speak many syllables fluently on one breath. Through constant vigilance and practice, this fluency technique is then maintained.

THE EDINBURGH MASKER

The Edinburgh masker, designed by Dr and Mrs Dewar, is one of the most recent appliances designed to alleviate stammering. It is a small, portable, electronic device consisting of ear moulds, like those used for hearing-aids, a small microphone attached at the level of the larynx with velcro tape, and a control box that can be placed in a pocket.

It has been known for some time that if speech is 'masked' so that the speaker cannot hear himself speak stammering is greatly reduced or totally eliminated. With the Edinburgh masker, as speech commences the throat microphone is activated by movement of the larynx and a loud, continuous tone is transmitted through the earpieces to both ears. As long as the wearer is talking the tone continues, so that the speaker cannot hear himself speak. When he stops talking the tone also stops.

The masker is suitable only for adults and is intended for use after conventional therapy has proved unsuccessful. It is essential that a speech therapist's advice is sought, as this device works only for some people, and it is necessary to have instruction on how to handle it in the most effective way.

The advantages of the masker are that some stammerers can be totally fluent whilst wearing it, and that the speaker has to make little effort to achieve fluency. Disadvantages are that it does not work for everyone; that many people find it difficult to tolerate the loud tone in their ears every time they speak; and that the speaker is dependent on the device for his fluency and, like all mechanical gadgets, it can break down.

Some therapists feel that the masker is useful in helping severe stammerers to learn a fluency technique and to acquire some experience of speaking fluently. When this has been achieved the device is worn less and less. It has also been found helpful for some clients on important occasions when fluency seems essential, for example when making a speech or an important telephone call.

To obtain the Edinburgh masker a medical referral is required and/or a letter from a speech therapist. It is available privately at a cost of about £110 or under the N.H.S. from the manufacturers, whose name and address is given on page 118.

THE HECTOR SPEECH AID

The Hector Speech Aid has recently been invented by two men who themselves stammer. The Aid consists of a pocket-sized control unit wired to a neckband, supporting a throat-microphone and a speaker. Speech is relayed by the microphone to the control unit which calculates the wearer's speech rate. When the wearer speaks too quickly the control unit transmits a tone – the volume of the tone can be adjusted. As the wearer slows his speech down the warning tone fades.

It is known that many people who stammer can become more fluent if they are able to slow down their speaking rate – indeed, an important factor in the technique of slow-prolonged speech is slowing down (see p. 78). The inventors of HECTOR found that, in everyday situations, they were unable to maintain the high rate of fluency they had achieved in speech therapy classes. Initially they designed this Aid to act as their personal speech-rate monitor. It proved so helpful that it has now been marketed to assist others to speak with more control and confidence by prompting them not to speak too quickly. HECTOR is only useful for those speakers who feel that too fast a rate of speech plays a part in their stammering problem.

The advantage of HECTOR is that it is under the speaker's control. It is his decision when to wear it, when to switch it on or off, and to what speed it is set. It is a teaching aid and not an instant cure. HECTOR costs approx. £150 and is available direct from the manufacturers' address p. 118.

'STAMMER MORE FLUENTLY' APPROACHES

Descriptions of the work of Charles Van Riper and Joseph Sheehan will give the reader an idea of the focus of treatment using the 'stammer more fluently' approach, as most other therapists base much of their treatment on the work of these two authorities.

CHARLES VAN RIPER'S TREATMENT

In his book *The Treatment of Stuttering* Van Riper devotes over 200 pages to his treatment and the following description is necessarily condensed.

The method is based on Van Riper's conviction that a stammerer does not need to be taught how to speak fluently as he can already do this. That may seem an absurd statement, but it is based on considerable evidence. Most people who stammer produce rather more fluent words than stammered words in their total speech output; also, a man may go into a shop and ask for a 'b – b – b –box of mmmmmmatches' and yet a short time later when sitting by himself at home he will be able to say 'box of matches' with both ease and fluency. It would seem that most stammerers *can* speak fluently, but that the fluency breaks down in certain circumstances.

The rationale behind this treatment is that there is no necessity to teach the stammerer to speak fluently as he already knows how to do this, but there is a necessity to teach him to cope with his feelings about stammering and with the actual stammer when it occurs. In this way, the client, instead of finding himself helpless as he anticipates or experiences stammering, learns to take charge and control his speech.

Van Riper describes treatment procedures within the four phases of his therapy:

1 *The Identification Phase* The client and therapist look closely at exactly what the client *does* when he stammers because it is difficult to change a pattern of behaviour if the true nature of that pattern is not known. When saying the word 'part', one man may get stuck on the 'p' sound and push hard until the word virtually explodes out of his mouth; another may begin to block on the 'p' sound and stop, go back to the previous word or phrase and try

to take a run into the word; yet another man may feel he is going to block and so insert a different sound, so that he ends by saying 'er, er, er, part'. This identification phase of treatment is also linked to the belief that facing the unfaceable and touching the untouchable helps to reduce the client's fear as he begins to look at his stammer and break it down to manageable proportions.

2 *The Desensitisation Phase* This is geared towards reducing speech fears and other feelings that may have developed around stammering, such as guilt, embarrassment, anger, and so on. Some stammerers are so disturbed by moments of stammering that they are unable to enjoy a life overshadowed by their speech difficulties. The client is helped to become less upset, to accept some degree of stammering in his speech and to appreciate that not everyone judges him as harshly as he judges himself. Once stammering becomes less of a focal point for feelings and emotions, it is possible to work on the actual speech problem.

3 *The Modification Phase* This involves dealing with the moment of stammering. The client is encouraged to change the way he has always stammered, and to reduce the struggle and avoidance behaviour. In this way, a more fluent and less abnormal stammering pattern is established. The emphasis is still on 'stammering fluently'. For example, if the client says 'part' by inserting 'er, er, er', this is abnormal because while saying 'er' he cannot say 'part' – it is impossible to have two different sounds in the mouth at the same time. In order to say 'part', it is essential to make the right contact for a 'p' sound and then move on to the next sound. Going back to take a run at a word – for example by inserting 'well, you see' – is abnormal because speech is an ongoing process, moving forwards from one sound to the next and one word to the next. Going back within a word is also abnormal. When saying 'su–su–su–supper' the speaker is going backwards, away from the feared 'p' sound, instead of towards it. During this phase, although the client will still stammer, he learns to use the sounds that he wishes to say and to get his speech moving forwards.

4 *The Stabilisation Phase* The client is helped to practise and use his new, fluent pattern of stammering. He must remain vigilant so that old fears and habits do not return, and his relaxed, gentle stammering pattern is retained. Slowly but surely, the client will walk the road towards fluency as his fears fade and his stammer reduces.

JOSEPH SHEEHAN'S TREATMENT

Sheehan thinks that treatment should start with work on some hidden features of stammering, and not directly on fluency. He believes it is essential that, through discussion and exercises, the therapist helps the client in the following ways:

To reduce the client's need to avoid stammering   Although some adult stammerers avoid rarely, many have developed the habit of hiding their stammer, and creating an illusion of fluency by keeping away from certain sounds, words, situations or people. It is thought that the more the client avoids stammering the more he increases his fear of stammering. The more he fears stammering, the more he will stammer – so that he is caught in a vicious circle. A man who stammers severely and frequently will have obtained his job with the employer's full knowledge that he stammers; he has made friends while stammering; his family accept him as a man who stammers. Conversely, another man who is extremely fluent by dint of hiding and avoiding his stammer may feel increasing anxiety as promotion at work becomes possible because, if he stammers, he may lose this promotion; if he stammers, his fiancée might call off the engagement; if he stammers, his friends may no longer like him. This man has built his life on avoidance and pretence, and his anxieties increase as he sees himself losing all he has achieved if anyone discovers that he stammers. The fear that grows from hiding and avoiding stammering is far greater than the fear when stammering actually occurs. Therefore a considerable amount of work is directed towards encouraging the client to allow his stammer to be seen and heard, to allow it to come into the open. Gradually the need to avoid and hide will be reduced, together with the fears of speaking.

To help the client to accept himself as a stammerer   An adult client may spend much of his time pretending that he is not a stammerer. He plays the part of a fluent person and refuses to accept himself as a stammerer. This constant pretence creates anxiety, conflict and tension, and Sheehan states that the more the client strives to behave like a fluent person, the more he will stammer because he is putting himself under so much pressure; the more he accepts himself as a stammerer, the more fluent he will become because he has lifted the pressure and is free to be himself. The stammerer is helped towards this acceptance through discussion and various speech tasks.

To teach the client more normal phrasing and pausing in speech The reasoning here is that many stammerers fear silence and pauses in speech and if these aspects are taught the fear will be reduced. (Pausing and normal flow or phrasing are also taught as part of the slow/prolonged technique. This is one example of how the two major approaches overlap. The aims differ. Sheehan's aim is to reduce the client's fears of silence so that he gains confidence in being able to stop talking and start again; the aim with slow/prolonged speech is to teach the client a more normal, fluent speaking pattern.)

The primary aim of Sheehan's treatment procedures is to help in reducing the client's fear – fears of stammering, of being a stammerer, and of what other people think. By decreasing his need to hide, avoid and pretend, the stammerer gradually increases his confidence in speech and his relationships with people around him.

OTHER METHODS

There is little doubt that almost any procedure will be successful for some people, but unless there is evidence that many people have obtained long-term benefits all that can be said is that the treatment has proved successful for a few clients. A stammerer once said that he had heard of a marvellous 'cure', which consisted of taping a small, metal disc to the scalp under the hair. This procedure had apparently 'cured' his friend. The friend may well have become fluent, but it is obvious that few adult stammerers would benefit similarly.

In evaluating the following methods of treatment, it is necessary to distinguish between a treatment that is used on its own and the same treatment when used in conjunction with speech therapy.

HYPNOSIS

There are difficulties in assessing the contribution of hypnosis to stammering therapy. Most hypnotists who have worked with stammerers and found their treatment successful do not give adequate information. For example, they do not describe the type of stammer, the feelings of the client, the suggestions given under hypnosis, or for how long the client remained fluent. Hypnosis as the sole form of treatment seems to have been effective for a few clients, but there is little knowledge of why it was effective. Was it something in the client, something about the stammer or a special technique used by the hypnotist?

However, there is some evidence that when speech therapists work together with a hypnotist, each providing specialised skill and knowledge, the approach has sometimes proved successful. The main drawback is that there is a shortage of qualified hypnotists, and so this joint approach is rarely possible. Although the idea of alleviating stammering through hypnosis is extremely attractive, it must be said that the success rate does not seem high.

RELAXATION, YOGA, MEDITATION

It has long been found that when the client is extremely relaxed the severity and frequency of stammering are reduced. The problem is for the client to maintain the feeling of relaxation when he is outside the safety of the clinic. Results when relaxation is the sole form of treatment are not encouraging. However, many speech therapists incorporate some form of relaxation work into their total treatment plan, and many clients find this helpful. With a greater ability to control physical tension, the client finds it easier to concentrate on the treatment procedures he is learning, and to use these in his everyday life.

I know of no reports of the use of yoga or meditation in stammering therapy, but have known several clients who have worked on these methods and found them advantageous. It may well be that a person who feels generally tense and anxious is prepared to spend the time and effort needed and so attains a calmer and more peaceful attitude to life in general and stammering in particular.

These kinds of treatment seem to work on relaxing the client, rather than creating any long-term cure of his stammer. However, when more relaxed, people are often physically healthier and mentally more alert. In this state, they are better able to cope with the stresses and tensions of living, and so become less sensitive about stammering and more able to use the speech techniques they have learnt.

MEDICINES

The most usual medicines prescribed by doctors are sedatives or tranquillisers, which will help to calm a patient complaining of feeling anxious and worried. It is essential to differentiate between a patient who is diagnosed by his doctor as being highly anxious and likely to benefit from these medicines and a patient who is given these medicines for the sole purpose of helping his stammer.

The treatment of stammering by the use of sedatives and tranquillisers is rarely successful and has the added drawback that, even if the patient becomes more fluent whilst on a course of pills, he must eventually stop taking them. Some clients actually stammer more severely when taking these medicines because they feel rather drowsy and are unable to concentrate fully.

PSYCHOTHERAPY

Psychotherapy is a very wide field and it is difficult to make any general statement on its value in the treatment of stammering, but the following points are worth considering.

- Sheehan states that 'To say that stutterers need psychotherapy or can profit from it is like saying people need psychotherapy or can profit from it'. Stammerers, as a group, have neither more nor fewer emotional problems than fluent speakers – except that they usually have some degree of anxiety associated with the stammer. Some fluent people require psychotherapy and so do some stammerers but the mere fact that someone stammers does not mean he either needs or will benefit from psychotherapy.
- The general term 'psychotherapy' includes a vast range of differing treatment approaches to deal with psychologically based problems. Some of these treatments may be beneficial to some stammerers, but no treatment method will be beneficial to all stammerers.
- It is impossible to draw a neat dividing line between psychotherapy and speech therapy. Psychotherapists and speech therapists use certain treatment methods which they have in common, but each is a specialist in her own field. A speech therapist is trained to deal specifically with speech and language problems, whilst a psychotherapist's training enables her to deal with emotional and behavioural problems not specifically related to speech. Many speech therapists working with adult stammerers use psychotherapeutic methods in their treatment – particularly when dealing with feelings and attitudes which have developed around the stammer. Some psychotherapists have specialised in speech problems and are able to help the client through psychotherapy, but also with methods used by speech therapists.

There is certainly a place for psychotherapy in the treatment of adult stammerers. Whether the ideal form of treatment is from a speech therapist with knowledge of psychotherapy or from a psychotherapist with knowledge of speech therapy cannot be established. Much will depend on the individual client, the nature of his stammer and the skills of the therapist involved.

PERSONAL CONSTRUCT PSYCHOTHERAPY

Some speech therapists are now studying and working with a particular psychotherapeutic approach called personal construct psychotherapy – a theory developed by the American psychologist George Kelly. The treatment is based on the belief that fluency, however desirable, is often a strange and unfamiliar world to the stammerer. It is possible that some clients do not maintain fluency because they cannot cope with all the new experiences that fluency brings. An important part of this therapy is to help the client develop his ideas about what it is like to be fluent and about himself as a person. Further information may be obtained from: The Centre for Personal Construct Psychology, Therapy and Counselling (address on page 118).

SUMMARY

If you are apprehensive about starting therapy, or if you feel you have gone as far as you can with your present therapy, consider, in the light of the information given in this chapter, whether a different approach or technique would suit you better at the stage you have now reached. If therapy for the confirmed stammerer is to be successful, all must travel hopefully, work at it, and be prepared to change direction – therapists and clients alike.

Chapter 12

Helping Yourself

Details of specific self-help books are given on p. 116. They are well worth reading. Each book contains its own advice, but there are common themes and you must find the path that is most useful to your needs.

This chapter is written not as a substitute for other books but to give my own views on this subject and to allow the reader who is eager to make a start to consider some steps immediately.

There is practical advice which will help you to change and improve your speech, and advice which may help you to re-evaluate your attitude to stammering and communication. From the ideas listed below you should select those suggestions that are most relevant to you as a person and for your stammer.

TACKLING YOUR STAMMER IS GOING TO BE HARD WORK

It seems unfair that most people can speak without worry or trouble, whilst others have to strive to achieve control. However, the first step on the road to mastering your speech is to accept that this will be hard work, requiring considerable stamina and dedication. You have already made a start by deciding to read this book, and can now begin travelling along the road towards greater fluency and control.

YOU DO NOT HAVE TO BE FLUENT ALL THE TIME

A client has asked me to devote a whole chapter to this statement as he feels that, when he began to understand it, his whole life changed. This may not be true for you, but there is little doubt that many stammerers see only two possibilities – to stammer or to be totally fluent. With this thought ever present in his mind, no matter how fluent a man may become, as soon as this fluency is interrupted by a stammer he feels that he is back to square one. When you accept that you do not have to be fluent 100 per cent of the time, and that the occasional stumble does not make you a permanent stammerer, life does become easier. You then begin to think of yourself as a fluent person who occasionally stammers rather than a stammerer who is occasionally fluent. Once you can think of yourself in this way, you will not need to struggle and become tense when you stammer, but will accept the stammer as a momentary interruption in your fluent speech.

LOOK AT WHAT YOU DO WHEN YOU STAMMER

Chapters 9 and 10 contain questionnaires to help you identify fairly precisely what you do when you stammer. Do not avoid this task. You need to be able to face your stammer, to become familiar with it and to break it up into manageable parts. Use a mirror and tape recorder as an aid and try to decide what you do that is different from normal speech and interferes with it. Work at reducing one abnormal pattern at a time and start by aiming to *change* that pattern rather than eliminating it. First, consider whether you have any unusual movements associated with your stammer, such as clenching your hand, putting your head down or tapping your foot. For example, you may find that you put your head down nearly every time that you stammer; attempt to change this head movement by putting your head backwards or sideways instead. This may seem a very strange suggestion, but it is difficult to change a mannerism radically in one step – to go from putting the head down to keeping it in a normal position. It is more effective to vary the movement until the original habit is weakened and then proceed to the final goal – in this case a normal head position. In a recent group one young man always rubbed his nose with his right forefinger just before he stammered. In order to change this movement which had become associated with his stammer, the man chose to try to rub his nose with his left forefinger for the next few days. By the time he returned the following week this particular mannerism had been so weakened that it was virtually eliminated – the stammer was no longer linked with a movement of left or right forefinger.

It is important to differentiate between movements which are natural and easy and those which are always associated with stammering and have become a part of the stammer. As you gain control over these movements, you can progress to changing abnormal movements directly connected with speech. Perhaps you often open your mouth when starting to block on a word; if so, begin to change this mouth movement and aim at making the appropriate contact for the sound you want to say. Do not aim at fluency at this stage, but work towards stammering in a more appropriate way using normal speech movements and normal speech contacts. For example it is unnecessary to rub your nose in order to say 'b'; it is impossible to say 'b' (requiring contact or touching of the lips) whilst your mouth is open; therefore, it must be helpful to aim at using natural hand movements and at putting the lips together gently because then, although still stammering, you are in the correct position for normal speech.

SLOW DOWN AND SPEAK MORE SLOWLY

Many stammerers feel a need to rush at speech and so speak at too fast a rate most of the time, or in bursts of speed when anticipating or experiencing a stammer. For many people, when the rate of speech is slowed down, the inner feelings of panic and urgency are reduced, and it becomes easier to handle the stammer. If you are interested in the slow/prolonged speech technique mentioned in Chapter 11, a cassette tape demonstrating and describing this method plus an information leaflet is available from the Association for Stammerers at a cost of £2·95, including postage.

SLOW DOWN AND STAMMER MORE SLOWLY

It is not only the speaking rate when fluent which should be slowed down, but the actual moment when you stammer. Trying to hurry through increases feelings of fear and may break up the natural rhythm involved in normal speaking. Slowing down the stammer as well as the fluent speech increases control so that you begin to have a sensation of taking charge of your speech instead of your speech being in charge of you.

TAKE ONE STEP AT A TIME

The changes you make will be successful and permanent only if they are taken slowly and patiently. Taking a run at fluency can end in disappointment. Sit down and make a careful plan for yourself. If, for instance, you decide to make a start by slowing down your whole speaking rate so that you not only speak more slowly but also stammer more slowly, then begin by practising when you are alone – preferably using a tape recorder to check what you are doing. Set yourself a target of perhaps three minutes, three times per day, when you will read into the recorder slowly and easily until you have gained some experience and confidence; then increase the reading to five and ten minutes, two or three times per day.

Often a client will say, 'There is little point in this exercise because I am always fluent when I'm by myself.' Most people are fluent when by themselves, but the purpose of this exercise is to practise a slow, easy form of speech in a relaxed atmosphere so that you can experience and feel the changes that occur without interruption or pressure from others.

Only when you feel comfortable and familiar with this pattern of speaking are you ready to progress from reading to talking. Sit by yourself and talk into the tape recorder for three minutes. Describe the room in which you are sitting, describe a holiday you have had or a film you have seen, and so on. Extend this period of talking, and keep checking what you are doing on your tape recorder. When you have become accustomed to talking in a slower manner when by yourself, move on to having a short conversation with one other person. Choose a member of your family or a friend to whom you can explain what you are doing, and again confine yourself to just a few minutes per day – only gradually increasing the period of time until you can talk to this other person for fifteen minutes, speaking more slowly and stammering more slowly. It may take several weeks of this step-by-step practising before you are ready to use your new type of speech in other situations. Choose a situation in which you feel at ease. Try your slow speaking and stammering for just a few minutes. Increase the time slowly. Set yourself goals which you can reach, rather than aiming at long periods of speaking, which may end with feelings of failure and frustration. Plan how to proceed day by day, using the slower form of speech or working on changing abnormal general and speech movements for increasing periods of time, but only in situations that are generally easy for you. Not until this has been accomplished will you be in a position to use the changed speaking pattern in more difficult situations. Set yourself realistic aims because, each time you succeed, you will have taken another step on the road. If you attempt to do too much too quickly you may continually fail and little is achieved.

This step-by-step procedure is important for every speaking task you decide to undertake, and it may help to remember two aspects, which can influence your speech – the person to whom you are speaking and the content of what you are saying. If you believe that your listener poses a threat of some kind, is judging you, is critical or authoritarian – then this may disrupt your speech. Therefore always start by choosing a listener who does not pose this kind of threat. Secondly, if the content of what you are saying is extremely important or very precise this too may influence your speech, so begin by talking about easy, general subjects.

RESIST TIME PRESSURE

It is important that you resist the need to hurry through speech in order not to bore or inconvenience other people. When talking to clients, I am frequently reminded of my friend Ann, who never wanted to drive a car. As her husband obtained promotion, he was given a company car and so the family vehicle stood outside the front door as Ann walked to work, to the shops and about her business. Finally, her family and friends persuaded her to learn to drive. Ann took countless lessons and eventually entered for her test. It took five tests before she obtained a licence and, with some trepidation, went for her first drive as a qualified but nervous driver. Ann lives in a wide, suburban street and, that morning, she drove along this street with her heart thumping. Looking in the mirror, she saw a van approaching at some speed, obviously intent on overtaking her. Ann panicked, decided she must give the van the right of way, attempted to draw into the side of the road and succeeded in mounting the pavement, hitting a tree and smashing the front of the car. The van driver carried on unperturbed. A confident driver would have looked into the mirror, registered the van approaching and left it to the van driver to decide whether to slow down or overtake.

Perhaps, like Ann who felt convinced that she must give way to more competent drivers, you have the feeling that you must give way to fluent speakers during a conversation. You feel under time pressure, and responsible if the listener shows any signs of impatience. Many fluent speakers talk slowly and take their time, and you should consider seriously whether or not you believe that you have the same rights as a fluent speaker. Take for example the situation when there is a queue of people behind you and you become worried because you believe that you are taking too long buying your ticket as you have no right to keep people waiting. If someone in that queue is in a desperate hurry, why is that your responsibility? What if a fluent speaker behind you takes several minutes over a lengthy inquiry about a season ticket – the inquiry will be made regardless of whether anyone is waiting. Just as it was up to the van driver to make his own decision, so it may be up to an impatient person to make her decision. Why did she not reach the ticket office with sufficient time to wait? Why does she show such impatience? You have just the same rights as fluent speakers. Do not allow other people's impatience or hurry to affect you. Resist time pressure – you may be surprised to find that, if you keep calm, others will calm down with you.

GO FORWARDS

Normal speech is essentially a forward-moving process – from one sound to the next and from one word to the next. Going back, taking a run into a word, trying to say the same sound over and over again is contrary to normal speaking. Set yourself short periods of time when you deliberately go forwards – however stuck or blocked on a sound you may feel. Choose a goal of perhaps two or three words per day, and then gradually increase this goal. On those two or three words, go forwards from sound to sound with as little struggle and tension as possible. Do not aim to say the word fluently. However much you stammer, aim to go on to the next sound and the next until the word is said. For example, when saying 'potato', if you get blocked on the 'p' at the beginning, do not repeat that sound, p–p–p–p–p–, as this is going backwards; once you have said the 'p', try to move on to 'o', 't', and so on, until you have moved forwards through the word 'potato'. This will help to give you a feeling of normal speaking, even though you may be stammering.

LOOK AT PEOPLE

If you often look away, close your eyes or blink when you stammer, this is a part of the stammer and adds strength to it and keeps it going. Try to look at the listener when you stammer and you will begin to feel much freer and less afraid. Closing the eyes or looking away when speaking is not natural and changing this behaviour will make your speech more normal. Obviously, you do not want to go to the opposite extreme of staring at the listener throughout an entire conversation but, during moments of stammering, you should increase your ability to keep your eyes open and look at others.

LOOKING AT THE WORLD AS A STAMMERER

Let me explain in this way: apparently, the Eskimos have

approximately 200 words to describe snow. Many of us are at a loss to find more than ten words to describe snow and, as one client said, 'That's because the Eskimos are up to their ears in snow and surrounded by snow.' Exactly the point I would like to make. Presumably an Eskimo spends much of his life surrounded by snow, dependent on snow and concerned with the condition of the snow. This analogy seems to apply to many stammerers. You may feel that you are up to your ears in stammering and surrounded by stammering without being able to appreciate that the majority of fluent speakers do not share your experiences or your concern. Certainly, most fluent speakers notice the moment of stammering, but this is a fleeting awareness, and is often unaccompanied by any feelings or judgement on the part of the listener. The fluent speaker has none of the experiences of the stammerer; he believes that stammering equals the moments when stammering occurs and is unaware of your feelings and fears because he has none of your experiences. It is important not to focus your own feelings onto the fluent listener and imagine that because you feel embarrassed he feels embarrassed, and because you feel anxious he feels anxious. The listener has his own problems and experiences – he may be far more concerned about his promotion prospects or his financial difficulties than about whether or not you stammer.

TRY NOT TO FIGHT OR HIDE YOUR STAMMER

Many stammerers try to hide and avoid their stammer because they are certain that fluent speakers share their thoughts about stammering – that it is embarrassing, humiliating, foolish, annoying, and so on. Perhaps it will help to keep thinking about the Eskimos in order to realise that fluent speakers have not lived your life and are not up to their ears in stammering nor are they surrounded by it. The term 'fluent speakers' covers a vast range of different people. Some will be intolerant of all kinds of behaviour, including stammering; others will be indifferent to such aspects as how a person looks or speaks if that person is pleasant. You cannot assume that all or even most listeners will react adversely to stammering, so begin to look at your speech more objectively and take account of the fact that others will view your speech as one part of you, and not as the whole of you.

If, for a long period of time, you have felt that it is essential for your life and well-being to hide your stammer from others, it will be hard to change this attitude. The fact remains that the harder you try to hide and avoid the more you will increase inner anxiety and the greater will be the tension when the stammer occurs. Again, set yourself small goals – perhaps two words in one day, when you will allow the stammer to come out into the open and try to tackle it slowly, going forward with as little tension as possible. It may seem ridiculous to let the stammer happen when you have hidden it successfully for so long; yet, if you found it helpful to hide your stammer and were happy with this method, you would not be reading this book. There is no easy path – you cannot hide your stammer and decrease your fears at the same time. Allow the stammer to emerge slowly and easily just a few times, and your fears will lessen as you find that listeners are rarely as concerned or bothered as you had imagined. What seemed to you a cataclysmic event has gone almost unnoticed. You cannot know until you try. Your fears may be imaginary because you see everything from the stand-point of the stammerer, and the fluent person sees it differently.

LISTEN TO HOW FLUENT PEOPLE SPEAK

In order to help change the feeling that either you are a stammerer or you are fluent, make a point of listening closely to how so-called fluent speakers really speak. Listen on buses and in trains; if you live in an area where there are phone-in programmes on the radio, tape record such a programme and then listen to the amount of 'fluent' speech you hear. You will discover that fluent people often have many hesitations in their speech, but they do not react to this disfluency. Few people are able to express their thoughts clearly and efficiently at all times; most people hesitate, repeat sounds and words, and insert 'you know' and other phrases to give themselves time to think. Some people are certainly highly fluent, but there are others who sound as though they are stammering, but appear totally unaware of and unconcerned at their disfluency. Learn to become more realistic about 'fluent' speech so that you cease to judge each moment of stammering as a disaster, and recognise that most people have some degree of disfluency in their speech.

A man was working on allowing his stammer to come into the open without struggle and avoidance. He found this extremely difficult but, after many weeks, decided to spend one whole morning aiming to stammer freely. On the morning he had chosen for this Herculean task, he went to the bank where he worked and, as he sat down to wait for his first customer, he heard the bank clerk sitting next to him say, 'D–d–d–did you want five or t–t–ten pound notes, sir?' This bank clerk was not practising his speech, did not have a stammer, nor was he aware of the slight repetitions. He had had a very late night, was tired and naturally hesitating. It was a lucky occurrence because it gave our man a little extra courage to begin his task, and he did very well that morning by allowing his stammer to flow quite easily out of his mouth. Although he had these easy repetitions more frequently than the 'fluent' clerk sitting next to him, the quality of their speech was much the same, as neither of them struggled with speech. One was aware of what he was doing and why, the other was not. To the customers there was probably little difference.

LISTEN ATTENTIVELY

You may find that you have spent so much time being concerned with how and when you can speak that it is quite difficult for you to listen. It is not just a question of listening to how others speak but, more important, to what they are saying. Although other speakers may be more fluent, they are still talking because they want to convey their thoughts and feelings and have them understood. If you become too involved in your own speech, you may antagonise the other person in a conversation, not because you stammer but because you do not appear to listen. It often helps considerably to set yourself the task of truly listening for a specified period of time – say five minutes. During those minutes, concentrate on what the speaker is trying to convey to you, how he is feeling and what he wants from you. I am reminded of Joan, who told me that she became silent and worried when a friend began to discuss her small child, who was not doing well at school. Joan had no children of her own and felt she had nothing to contribute to this conversation, even had she been fluent. As a stammerer, she had even less. Yet, in this situation, the most likely need of the speaker was to find some-one who would listen calmly and with understanding to her worries about the child. Perhaps the occasional nod or muttered 'I see. Oh dear' might have been called for, but it is unlikely that a deep knowledge of education or excellent speaking skills were required. Joan was so enclosed by her own feelings of inadequacy, as a person with little experience of children and as a speaker with little experience of fluency, that she felt unable to contribute the one thing that was probably needed – being a good listener. Develop your listening skills and you will find yourself more interested in others, more aware of them as individuals with their own joys and sorrows, and less focused on just one thing – your stammer.

FEEL AND EXPERIENCE YOUR OWN FLUENT SPEECH

Many stammerers have a good deal of fluent speech in their overall speaking yet often this fluent speech is forgotten and dismissed whilst stammered words are given undue attention and importance. I recall a client who attended a class one evening at 7 p.m., and informed the assembled group that he had had a 'terrible' day. When questioned, he revealed that he had gone to the station that morning at 8.30 a.m. and asked for a ticket to 'Fenchurch Street'; he had found himself totally blocked on 'Fenchurch' and felt he spent several minutes struggling to say this word. It had been a 'terrible' experience and left him dispirited and depressed. We asked what had happened since this episode – between 8.30 a.m. and our meeting at 7 p.m.? He seemed surprised by the question, considered it for a moment, and then said: 'Oh, I've been all right since then – it was saying "Fenchurch Street" that was so terrible.' This man had apparently been quite fluent all day and yet the one distressing moment, first thing in the morning, so preoccupied him that the rest of the day was dismissed and the fluency neither noted nor considered.

Value your fluency, experience your fluency, become aware of what it feels like when you speak fluently. If you are only truly aware of the moments of stammering, you cannot work on extending your fluency as you have paid insufficient attention to the sensations you experience when fluent, and to how your mouth, lips, tongue and speech organs move and behave when you are fluent as opposed to when you are stammering.

TALK ABOUT STAMMERING

Another aid in not avoiding or hiding the stammer is to start to talk about it more openly. Many people will not broach the subject unless you start the conversation. You may feel that it is pointless to talk about stammering to your family, friends and colleagues as they are aware that you have a stammer. Doubtless they do know that you stammer, but the important issue is that you need to be more open about the subject and not believe that everyone is centred on your stammering, or particularly interested in it. Once you start to talk about stammering, about what you are doing to help yourself, what it feels like to stammer, and how others can help you, you will be surprised how gradually the whole subject will assume less importance and be less central in your life.

WHAT ARE YOUR GOALS?

Ask yourself the question 'What do I want out of life?' and sit down to make a list of everything you want to achieve, feel, experience or obtain. Here is an example of a list from one client:

1 To be managing director of my company
2 To be admired
3 To be totally fluent
4 To be a great public speaker
5 To play football for Tottenham Hotspurs
6 A happy marriage
7 To have a family
8 To be rich
9 Not to be criticised
10 To be like Robert Redford

Now examine your list and try to establish which goals are reasonable and in the realms of possibility, and which goals are fairly unlikely. My client was happily married so point 6 was in his grasp; and, although not Robert Redford's twin, he felt sufficiently good looking to be near his goal 10. On the other hand, after several years of marriage, it had been established that this couple could not have children (point 7) and, as it can be destructive to self-confidence to continue striving towards a goal which is almost inaccessible, it was necessary to investigate whether this goal could be modified so it came within reach. In this instance, the possibility of adoption or fostering was discussed.

Try to be as precise as possible about what you mean by each goal. On point 3, the client was asked whether he meant total fluency, and it was found that he was willing to accept some disfluency providing he had no severe blocks, did not lose control over his speech and felt no agitation.

Look for any inconsistencies in your goals. For example, in the above list, it was thought that becoming managing director (1) and not being criticised (9) were probably incompatible. It is difficult to rise to the top in your work, be in charge and responsible for many people and complex decisions, and expect to play so safely that no one will ever criticise you. By listing his goals, my client was able to examine which of the two was most important – to get to the top or to avoid criticism.

List your goals in order of importance, and then plan clearly and precisely how to attain each important goal. It is not helpful to state that you want to be totally fluent as this is an unattainable goal for anyone, either fluent speaker or stammerer. It is more useful to specify that you want to stop having hard blocks in your speech. Most productive of all is to plan, for instance, to work on three blocks per day for one week so that by the end of that week you will be able to ease out of those three blocks per day with less struggle and tension. Equally, it is not very useful to aim at playing for Tottenham Hotspurs; it is more profitable to aim at playing for your local football team, but most helpful of all to aim at playing football once a week for the next six months so that you can test your fitness and ability and see more clearly how far you are able to go in the game.

Goals which are conflicting or virtually impossible to attain will cause anxiety and lessen your self-confidence. Attainable, manageable goals will increase your motivation and self-confidence.

The Chinese have a saying that a journey of a thousand miles starts with a single step. In reading this chapter, you have taken that single step. Let us hope that you will not need to cover one thousand miles before reaching your objectives, but that your work will bring its own rewards as you find yourself more fluent, happier and less tense because you are experiencing greater freedom of speech and greater confidence in speaking.

Chapter 13

From Those Who Stammer

Several of my clients suggested that I should include some accounts from those who stammer so that readers may be able to identify more closely with others who have had similar experiences or difficulties. The contributors were asked to supply any comments, experiences or advice which they felt might be useful for readers of this book. This chapter includes some of the replies received and I would like to thank everyone who was good enough to contribute. Unfortunately, space does not allow the inclusion of every contribution and I hope this will be forgiven.

Stammering is sometimes annoying and embarrassing but it doesn't matter too much. I do quite well at school and have lots of friends and I'm working at getting rid of my stammer, but don't spend much time thinking about it. My mum and dad say I should speak a bit more slowly and then I'll grow out of it. I expect I will grow out of it in about a year.

Alan, aged 11

The advice I would give to anyone reading this book is don't give up; don't feel sorry for yourself but find a way which helps you and work at it slowly, a bit day by day. Don't run away from your stammer, but develop a sense of humour and keep chipping away at it. You'll be all right.

John, aged 18

I don't like reading aloud in class, especially if I have to wait for a long time, but other than that my speech isn't too bad. Some weeks ago our teacher talked about people who wear glasses and things like that and he also talked about my speech. At first I was a bit embarrassed but then it was all right because we discussed it quite a lot. Malcolm, my best mate, wears glasses and that doesn't bother him so he doesn't see why I should bother about my stammer.

Mike, aged 13

I come here every week I think and we play games, but most of all I like painting and I do that at school too and I'm very good at painting. Sometimes we do music with the drum and clapping. I like coming here because there are lots of toys and best of all I like playing football at school and I watch it with my dad on telly.

David, aged 6

I have stammered a lot since I was quite young and I often feel so angry that I could punch someone. There are many times when I know what to say at home and at school but the words won't come out and then someone else starts speaking. I used to worry all the time, not just about the stammer and being different from the others at school but also about getting so mad and frustrated. I never wanted to see a speech therapist but I was sent about six months ago and at first I thought it was a real waste of time. Now I feel much better about things because she listens to me no matter how bad my stammer is and I'm a whole lot calmer when I'm with her. We work at slowing my speaking down and using light contacts and we talk about my getting angry. I think it will take a lot of time for my speech to come right but I don't feel as cut off as I used to.

Martin, aged 15

I had therapy when about 6 or 7 years, and then no more until after I left school and home and could have therapy without my parents knowing. My stammer was very rarely mentioned either at home or at school. It would have been less of a worry, I think, if it had been openly acknowledged that I did stammer and if I had received therapy to help me cope. Reading aloud was the main worry and some teachers eventually missed me out, which removed the fear of anticipation but didn't really help and I didn't like it. Some teachers would read aloud with me, which was slightly better.

When I was 19 years old I learnt syllabic speech and the relief it gave was miraculous and indescribable – being able to answer the phone, ask for train tickets, etc. Such was the motivation that for a while I wore an electric metronome in my ear and was sometimes taken for deaf. Prolonged/slowed speech came years later and again was very welcome and effective, although not quite the same miracle as I had never been so bad as in earlier times. I have attended group therapy evening classes and an intensive course and these have been fun and stimulating and have increased my confidence very much. Also, I have now reached a stage where, instead of thinking stammering is bad and shameful and must be controlled, I now feel it doesn't matter so much and am prepared to stammer gracefully through at least some blocks. At present I am very fluent but, although I know there will be ups and downs, I'm not too worried about the future.

Caroline, aged 32

One of the things that used to confuse me when I was at secondary school (I didn't notice it at junior school) was the different ways in which the various teachers coped with my stammer. Some would treat me like a normally fluent speaker while others would be 'kind' and miss me out when it came to my turn to read aloud. The lessons with the 'kind' teachers did not loom up like great big mountains, as did the other lessons, so I was able to concentrate more on the subject being taught, which probably helped me with my exam results.

In retrospect, I would come out in favour of the teachers with the harder approach because, although the 'kind' teachers may have helped me academically, they reinforced my stammer and my self-consciousness, making me feel slightly inferior and jealous of the other pupils. But how were those teachers able to recognise what stage my stammer had reached? Perhaps they should have talked about it, first with me and then, if appropriate, with the whole of the class.

Andrew, aged 39

From the listener's point of view I've always had a mild stammer, but that's not to say that for me it wasn't much of a problem. On the contrary, it became an enormous problem, so much so that in my early twenties I led a very negative life on account of the acute anxiety I suffered over my speech.

That is why I think having a 'mild' stammer really worked against me. Because I was able to pass as a normal fluent speaker most of the time it became for me a 'life-and-death issue' not to be caught out stammering. To avoid this and to maintain the pretence of being fluent, I built up over the years a very elaborate system of tricks and devices to cover up the fact that I was a stammerer.

Looking back now, it seems unbelievable the lengths I'd go to in order to avoid exposure. For years I avoided the phone, except in the most vital emergencies and thank God there weren't many of those.

Asking for cigarettes in shops wasn't a question of what brand I preferred but rather of which words I felt less inclined to stammer on.

Making bus journeys was another daily torture. I'd always try and make sure I had exactly the correct fare for the trip so I could just hand it over wordlessly. Failing that, I have been known to ask for a different destination from the one I really wanted if I felt this word would be less likely to precipitate a block, even if it involved walking a few extra hundred yards.

During a conversation, if I suddenly felt unable to say a particular word, one of my tricks was to simply pretend that I had forgotten what I wanted to say, and I'd 'um' and 'er' and look perplexed until I felt able to say it. I even did this sometimes after being asked my name and address. I need not add that I received some very odd looks. It's really a wonder I survived for so long without being 'carted off' in a yellow van.

As the years went by my fears and anxieties mounted; my avoidance behaviour grew ever more complex and my actual degree of natural fluency continued to decrease. I felt extremely isolated, because throughout all this time, right up until I was about 24 years old, I felt too ashamed to confide in anyone about this hang-up of mine – not even my parents or my husband! But even if I had felt able to discuss it with them it would have been impossible for them to appreciate how serious a problem my stammer was to me, as they were the very people that I could speak completely fluently with anyway.

Inevitably a crisis was reached, a breaking-point, where employing all my usual avoidance strategies wasn't enough to maintain my guise as a fluent speaker. With or without them it became more and more apparent that I was a stammerer. I had a choice: either come clean and seek therapy or take a vow of silence and become a recluse. I sought therapy.

Now, two years later, I have emerged from a very dark tunnel. Therapy for me has involved mainly a gradual, yet in the long term dramatic, change of attitude. I am far more confident and outgoing than I used to be and I now avoid very few speaking situations. But the best thing of all is that I've finally thrown off that ghastly sense of shame that I associated with stammering for fifteen very long years.

I feel like someone who is finally released from prison after serving a life sentence for a crime he didn't commit.

Elizabeth, aged 28

I started to stammer when I was 5 years old. From then until my marriage at 27 my stammer fluctuated between severe and very severe. It took the form of bad blocks accompanied by facial expressions and sometimes the waving of my arms – often with my head swaying from side to side. Strangely enough this caused little comment among my fellow pupils at school; it was not until I started work that I encountered rude and wounding comments from my elders and betters.

For the first year or so after leaving school I withdrew into myself, only speaking when spoken to, but gradually I learnt to ignore the remarks made to me and about me and gained enough confidence to lead a fairly normal life despite still having a serious speech problem.

By the time I met my wife-to-be, I had learnt to accept my impaired speech, or so I thought. When I was introduced to my wife's family I could not understand why there was a certain coolness towards me. Later when we got married their rejection of both my wife and myself was total and final. It was not until much later that I realised that I was both an embarrassment and a nuisance to them. It was then that I decided to have one final try at 'curing' my speech. It had shaped my life and had thrust me into jobs and situations that were not always suitable.

In my early forties I read an article in the *Sunday Times* that finally decided me to take the plunge. I little knew at the time the hard work and dedication that is needed to control, not cure, a stammer. Now, although I still stammer, my disfluency is much less and it no longer looms like a threatening black cloud over my life.

Incidentally, I refrain from talking to my wife's family!

Lionel, aged 45

My parents tell me that I started stammering about 3½ years old, but I was not really conscious of this until I was 7 or 8 years old and it didn't worry me till I was 10 or 11. It worried my parents, though, and it was they, and my sisters, who told me that I had a stammer. They had been told that if they ignored it it would go away, as my sister's stammer had, but it hadn't gone by the time I was 7 so I was sent to a speech therapist. Even though I was singled out from my class for the weekly visits to the speech therapist, and I knew I was different from the others because of my speech, the fact that I stammered did not bother me very much. I made my regular Tuesday afternoon trips to the clinic and this went on for a few years, but my parents could not see any marked improvement and so came to the conclusion (I don't know if the speech therapist had any say in this) that I did not know when I was stammering and so was not using the technique I'd been taught. I therefore had to be told when I was stammering so that I would know. I was then about 10 years old and I remember clearly my parents and sisters pulling me up time after time – 'Look, you're doing it now, you're doing it now.'

I don't blame my family for my present stammer – they were doing what they thought was best – but I do hold them responsible for pouring in the concrete that set so deep in me. My stammer didn't bother me, so why should it have bothered them?

Jonathan, aged 28

Imagine a quiet street in suburban Surrey about twenty years ago. Four telephone engineers have just alighted from their lorry which is parked beside a 20-foot telephone pole. The gang foreman has explained exactly what he requires of his team and I am amongst this brave body of men, a 20-year-old slip of a lad, as green as grass. 'Right-ho, laddie,' said the foreman, 'just shin up that pole and connect this portable telephone across line three. Contact the exchange engineer and ask him to test the line with you.' This was my maiden climb and my mind was racing ahead. For a start I am terrified of heights and the top of that pole seemed a long way up. Secondly, and to my mind a thousand times more terrifying, how on earth was I to get the message across with a stammer as bad as mine when the exchange engineer answered?

I strapped myself to the top of the pole and all went reasonably well until I heard the exchange engineer's voice and attempted to communicate with him. He had obviously never heard anything like this before. I was stammering very badly, gnashing and grinding my teeth, puffing and panting in my fruitless effort to speak. The poor engineer was so alarmed by this that he decided that I had actually fallen from the top of the pole and was in dire need of an ambulance. Down on the ground, the foreman eventually stopped laughing, composed himself and cancelled the ambulance. This then was my embarrassing, humiliating and painful initiation into the telephone service! One thing was certain – although I was completely fascinated by the theory and practicalities of the telephone system, my fear of actually using the damned thing was total and, as far as I could see, unconquerable.

Well, of course, time marches on and over the years I moved from department to department. In all this time my stammer did not improve and I developed all sorts of avoidance techniques, especially regarding the telephone. I would rather drive 10 or 20 miles to ask a question or deliver a message when I was surrounded by thousands of pounds worth of sophisticated telephone switching equipment! In the fullness of time the question arose as to whether or not I was potential management material. The British Post Office decides this question with a promotion board and I presented myself for this ordeal kitted out with the electronic Edinburgh masker – wired up for sound like some kind of robot and, because I could not hear myself speak every time the masker began to oscillate, shouting the answers at the top of my voice at the three interviewers across the table. At the conclusion, one of the good gentlemen inquired with one eye on the earphones attached to me, 'What is your problem, Mr X, are you deaf?'

Despite this comic performance, a management post was eventually offered to me. My moment of glory, the apex of my career, had finally arrived. Alas, what happened was just like a nightmare! My avoidance days were abruptly brought to an end as it dawned on me that a manager's job is to communicate by word of mouth. My new workplace was in an office with a couple of telephones that needed my constant attention. Imagine my absolute terror when my boss suggested that he would like me to contact Brighton HQ and ask a Mr B. B. about backward busying relay sets for Basingstoke Bounty Exchange. Need I say that my most feared words are those that start with a 'b'?

The game was up. I was in desperate need of help or else I was quite likely to go under. In fact, help was not far away and, like most things, it happened almost by chance – but that is another story. For the moment all I will say is that I spent a marvellous four weeks on an intensive speech therapy course at the City Lit. in London. My eyes and mind were opened to a whole new, wonderful world – a world of fluency in speech. Three gifted ladies helped me to start to piece together the long-lost rhythm of my voice and changed my life almost overnight.

When I returned to my office, I soon realised that I still had a long, long struggle ahead, but at last I had a point of reference. Despair had been replaced by hope and a growing confidence as I could feel the vicious cycle of stammering was being slowly dismantled. This was obviously going to be a long-term, very arduous project.

To come right up to date, my managerial duties now involve me in countless telephone calls, discussions, meetings and courses, all of which rely heavily on speech. It is still amazing to me that I am beginning to get immense enjoyment from these activities. Okay, minor setbacks do occur, but it must always be borne in mind that Rome wasn't built in a day. The sheer terror of the telephone is fading fast and it is rapidly becoming a useful friend that can save many hours of time. There will be people who will say that this transformation has probably come about simply as a side-effect of growing older, but this is not so. My stammer was getting worse and, at 36 years of age, I was becoming resigned to it. Speech therapy was indeed my saviour and my only regret is that it did not happen earlier. Within the past year I have learnt that a general slowing down of speech, prolongation of sounds, pausing, the awareness of hard and soft contacts on the initial consonant of a word and being able to take the urgency out of speech all help to unwind the vicious circle of stammering. However, all these weapons are useless if you cannot bring yourself to use them, especially when the going's rough. There must be a grim determination to succeed and perhaps a compelling reason to do so. I hate and loathe stammering and this is one hell of a reason for me to attempt anything to conquer it. I will admit that one must accept a certain amount of stammering, but it must be controlled and not the sort that freezes body and mind. Desensitisation to these terrible hidden effects of stammering is essential to a lasting 'cure'.

Recently it has occurred to me that when it comes to disabilities we stammerers are in some ways lucky because we know that there is nothing organically wrong with our speech mechanism as we can speak fluently at times. It would seem that, over the years, we have somehow taught ourselves to let our speech break down when tense, anxious and nervous situations threaten. I am convinced that what can be learned can be unlearned and a way can be found out of the dismal swamp of stammering. Certainly I do not underestimate the complex nature of this affliction. The fight is certainly not easy but, when a certain amount of success is achieved, it is soon realised that, by God, it is worth it!

Bernard, aged 36

I am 34 years old, married with two young children and I work as a computer consultant in London. From my experience, the advice I would give to fellow stammerers who have that 'if only I could cure my stammer' feeling is:

1 Try to obtain professional tuition/advice from a qualified speech therapist, however infrequently.
2 Try to be as open as possible about your stammer and discuss *positively* the ways in which you are tackling it.
3 Set up regular practice routines with planned progress milestones and remember your successes.

The advice I would give to speech therapists is that more attention should be focused on how a greater carry-over of fluency into the world outside the clinic can be achieved once the techniques have been mastered. Individual stammerers should be assisted in planning their own potential progress and then to measure achievement against that plan. In this way, weekly homework could be aimed at a particular goal or milestone rather than the vague target of fluency sometime in the future.

David, aged 34

Many people with mild stammers may not have sought speech therapy because they assume that the hard-pressed National Health Service will be obliged to devote all its limited resources to helping severe stammerers. My stammer has generally been mild, but to me it has been a constant source of anxiety and frustration. It has affected my confidence, my morale and my relationships with other people. Over the last few months, I have been both surprised and impressed by the quantity and quality of help provided by the therapists in the Health Service and the Inner London Education Authority. I would strongly urge mild stammerers to seek therapy if they are worried about their speech.

Speech therapy has been of great benefit to me in two particularly important ways. First, it has enabled me to gain very much greater fluency and control over my speech than ever before. Secondly, and probably of even greater significance, it has radically changed my previously negative attitude towards speech and stammering.

Speech therapy has introduced me to the slowed speech technique. In most situations my speech is now noticeably slower, smoother and more fluent. However, I would stress that a high degree of motivation and discipline is required by anyone learning the technique. Slowed speech is not a magic trick that can be learned in five minutes and turned on whenever stammering is anticipated. Before you decide to study the technique, you must accept that your present, habitual manner of speaking is inefficient and ineffective. You must also realise that it is difficult to change the bad habits of a lifetime. It has taken many months of constant practice to absorb the essential features of the technique into my speech. I am convinced that the effort has been well worth while.

The prospect of learning the slowed speech technique was rather alarming at first. I was worried that my speaking might become too mechanical and that other people would find me dreadfully boring! It is, however, not necesary to talk unduly slowly in real-life situations. As my speech has become slower and more fluent, my relationships with most other people have definitely improved. My speaking now comes over as being far more normal to others than my old stammering pattern of speech.

I have always been very sensitive about my stammer. At the merest hint of a minor hesitation I would say to myself, 'Help, I've stammered.' I would become tense and consequently I would probably stammer more. Stammering, to my mind, was degrading and I assumed that other people would think badly of me if they heard me stammer. Being so embarrassed about the subject, I hardly ever spoke to anyone about stammering and I had certainly never been able to admit that it caused me a great deal of worry and anxiety. For years I did everything possible to try and hide the unpalatable truth that I stammered, but the avoidance of words and situations merely served to heighten my frustrations. All my negative attitudes about stammering remained bottled up inside me.

Speech therapy has significantly reduced my sensitivity towards stammering. I now realise that far less notice was paid to my stammer than I'd imagined and that most people are very tolerant about stammering. Recently, I've discussed stammering and speech therapy with my friends, relatives and colleagues at work. Bringing the subject out into the open has given me a great sense of relief. No longer do I feel all alone with my problem and no longer do I feel under intense pressure to try and maintain perfect fluency at all times. Not worrying so much about stammering has enabled me to be more relaxed and confident with other people. As a result, I feel that I am communicating better than previously and stammering less.

John, aged 32

My first awareness of my stammer came at the age of about 5 when I noticed that responses from both parents and relations were becoming uncomfortable, and sometimes frightening. My mother would show intense anxiety, whereas my father would suddenly snap at me because (so I was told) I was stammering. Oddly enough I was rarely aware of these times myself, but this became clearer later on. Though I realise, of course, that family concern was shown with my own interests at heart, I was not aware of that at the time – the stammer was a problem I was utterly unable to resolve, I had no idea who to ask for advice, and I remember reactions at home to my stammer as being very unpleasant. They simply did not understand why I was having any difficulty. So I would suggest that, wherever possible, parents should be given some kind of advice about responding to the emergence of a stammer from their child (perhaps they are?) and try to avoid responding in negative ways, although of course it must put them under a lot of pressure.

Andy, aged 25

I feel that if the teachers at school had taken me aside and asked me how I felt about reading and general talking in front of a large group, it might have helped. I used to hate sitting in class waiting for my turn to come. The English teacher would either say in front of everyone 'Are you reading?' or just say 'We'll miss you out.' Perhaps the teacher should have said, 'Ann finds it difficult, but she likes to try.'

Ann, aged 31

Looking back over my thirty years as a stammerer, I reckon that the worst period was when I was thinking that I was getting the better of my stammer. My upper hand over it was hardly real, however, as so much anxiety still remained. In fact the anxiety was increased because my fluency was basically a cover-up job; to avoid serious blocking, which because of its rarity was all the more embarrassing when it happened, I had to avoid saying certain words. The mental energies that this little ploy required were enormous. The instantaneous editing process while speaking, having to substitute easy words for difficult ones, or having to rearrange sentences to enable me to get a lead in onto the difficult ones, taxed my brain and stretched my nervous system to its limits.

At this stage I never talked about my stammering to anyone and I felt very distressed about my position. Because of the success of my cover-up job, nobody realised that I simply had a stammer. My speech problem had become too complicated. How could I expect anyone to understand it? Outwardly I was just awkward and ill at ease and prone to be intense. Once I started talking I often couldn't stop. But none of these were problems that caused anyone to be concerned for me. No one knew how lonely I felt, how I dreaded the simplest talking situations, how unable I was to reach out naturally to people in conversation, or how hopeless I felt for the future.

In desperation I asked for help, something that only my pride had held me back from doing years before. And what a surprise! People were keen to help, and what a relief it was to me just to be able to talk about my problems. They shrunk to half their size as soon as I came clean about them. And there was a lot more help to come, as a result of which my speech has been coming back to normal.

I am still prone to stammer, but I am a much better communicator and very much happier for that. The old anxiety has practically disappeared.

Graham, aged 35

From *Speaking Out*

I was very impressed with the March edition and the article 'The Quest for Fluency' came as a breath of fresh air to me, as I had felt that my attitude towards my stammer was not correct and that I should be concentrating on 100 per cent fluency.

If I may indulge in telling the readers about my experience with stammering it will, perhaps, endorse the views in that article for those who are still sceptical.

After leaving school, the problem of stammering came to a head. Having left the relative protection of school, I now had to face the real world and all those speaking situations which are so hard to deal with. One day, while working in my father's shop, a lady came in and mentioned that her husband had a stammer and that he had gone to the City Lit. and was now almost 100 per cent fluent. On hearing this I wondered if this was a miracle cure, the one I had been looking for.

Some months later I set off for the City Lit. to be cured. On arrival we were met by a dynamic speech therapist who gave us a talk on the aims of the course: 'One thing we do not aim to do is to cure you; we can teach you how to control your stammer and how to deal with stressful situations, the rest is up to you.' On hearing this my heart sank – was there no cure?

The answer, as I now realise, is that your mental attitude towards your stammer can end up being your cure. On the City Lit. course I learnt some very valuable things about myself and other people. Stammerers are not the only people who find certain talking situations difficult, and not the only ones who find that they cannot get into certain jobs. If you think that if only you didn't have a stammer things would be different, it is a very unhappy way to carry on.

I now accept my stammer as part of my personality and do not aim for complete fluency, as I feel it is better to stammer a little and be happy than to always be struggling for a hopeless goal. The result of this attitude towards my stammer has resulted in it being less severe – an interesting thought!

I realise that there may be many of you reading this article who have a more severe stammer than mine. Of course you should try to reach a level of fluency with which you are happy. I think that this is my answer to stammering – reach a level of fluency that you are happy to live with.

Ron, aged 33

Suggested Reading

Controversies About Stuttering Therapy, edited by Hugo H. Gregory (University Park Press, 1979).
   Written by speech therapists for speech therapists this book has certain sections which will be of interest to readers seeking more academic information about therapy.

Stammering – Practical Help For All Ages, by Ann Irwin (Penguin, 1980).
   A self-help book giving general information about stammering as well as exercises for older children and adults based on this author's 'easy-stammering' therapy.

Overcoming Stammering, by R. M. MacDonald Ladell (A. Thomas & Co., 1973).
   A psychologist's view of the causes of stammering together with self-help methods for dealing with it.

Stammering Correction Simplified, by R. Muirden (J. Garnet Miller, 1971).
   This is a self-help book based on the author's own experience of how to overcome stammering.

Stuttering Solved, by Martin Schwartz (Heinemann, 1976).
   This is not a self-help book, but gives a description of Dr Schwartz's airflow technique together with general advice and information.

Speech Foundation of America Publications, P.O. Box 11749, Memphis, Tennessee 38111. These publications are available direct. Prices quoted do not include postage and packing and may well alter over a period of time.

Stuttering: Its Prevention (publication no. 3).
   Written by speech therapists for parents of very young children who are concerned about the child's speech. 50 cents.

To the Stutterer (publication no. 9).
   Written by 24 men and women speech therapists who are or have been stammerers, advising what helped them and what they believe will help others. $1·50.

If Your Child Stutters: A Guide For Parents (publication no. 11).
   Advice on what to do to help young stammerers of 3–6 years of age. 50 cents.

Self-Therapy for the Stutterer (publication no. 12).
   Written for the adult who is unable to take advantage of therapy. Outlines a self-therapy programme describing what the stammerer can and should do to tackle his problem and control his stammer. $2·50.

BOOKS OF GENERAL INTEREST

Living With Teenagers, by Tom Crabtree (MacDonald Futura, 1980).

Written by an educational psychologist to shed some light on the particular problems facing teenagers and their parents.

I'm O.K. – You're O.K., by Thomas A. Harris (Pan, 1973).

This book offers an approach to problem solving in general living and explains how to gain control of yourself, your relationships and your future – no matter what has happened in the past.

Inquiring Man, by D. Bannister and Fay Fransella (Penguin, 2nd edn 1980).

Personal construct theory is summarised in this book which lays emphasis on common human experience as the focus of psychology. It is not only aimed at students and psychologists, but could be of interest to anyone who is connected with or involved in working with people.

TAPE RECORDING

A tape recording and leaflet demonstrating and explaining the use of slow/prolonged speech is available from the Association for Stammerers, at £2·95 including postage.

Useful Addresses

UNITED KINGDOM

(This list not comprehensive. Therapists practise throughout the United Kingdom. It is important to seek out the facilities in your own area.)

The Association for Stammerers, 86 Blackfriars Road, London SE1 8HA. Will give information and help on all problems to do with stammering. May be able to put you in touch with other stammerers, in your area, with speech therapists or self-help groups. Membership fee £5 p.a. which includes free copies of quarterly journal *Speaking Out.* Will advise members and non-members.

The College of Speech Therapists, Harold Poster House, 6 Lechmere Road, London NW2 5BU. The professional body of speech therapists which can offer advice about NHS or private facilities for therapy in your area.

Mrs Lena Rustin (District Speech Therapist for Bloomsbury, Hampstead & Islington), Finsbury Health Centre, Pine Street, London EC1. Offers the following help for children under the NHS: consultation and advice for children aged 2½–7 years and their parents; intensive programmes in which parents are involved for 7–12 year-olds; intensive programmes for teenagers up to school-leaving age.

Speech Therapy Unit, The City Literary Institute, Keeley House, Keeley Street, London WC2B 4BA. Intensive day-time courses and weekly evening classes are offered for adults under the auspices of the ILEA. Those living outside London can usually be accepted on these courses. (Details of other ILEA classes for stammerers in London may be found in *Floodlight.*)

School for the Study of Disorders of Human Communication, 86 Black-friars Road, London SE1 8HA. Intensive courses are offered during some school holidays for children aged 11–17 years.

The Apple House, Warneford Hospital, Oxford. Short intensive courses for adults under the NHS.

Centre for Personal Construct Psychology Therapy and Counselling, 132 Warwick Way, London SW1 4JD. Private individual or group psychotherapy and counselling can be arranged.

Findlay, Irvine Ltd, Bog Road, Penicuick, Midlothian, Scotland. Manufacturers of the Edinburgh Masker.

Aleph One Ltd, PO Box No. 72, Cambridge CB3 0NX. Manufacturers of the Relaxometer, which is a biofeedback machine sometimes used as an aid in relaxation.

Peter Graham Partnership, 10 Eastway, Epsom, Surrey KT19 8SG. Tel: Epsom 23220. Manufacturers of the Hector Speech Aid.

When writing to the above organisations, please enclose stamped addressed envelope for early reply.

AUSTRALIA

Speak Easy Association (Peter Bartley), PO Box 156, Parramatta, New South Wales 2150

GERMANY

(There are many self-help groups throughout Germany, but only the one in Berlin is given here.)
Hans-Joachim Deckert, Gotzkowskistr. 4, 1000 Berlin 21

IRELAND (EIRE)

Irish Stammerers' Association (Tom Scally), Belvedere House, Belvedere Place, Dublin 1

JAPAN

Japanese Association for Stammerers for mutual help and friendship, Shinji Fukano, A–44–306 Khoro 5, Otokoyama, Yahata-shi, Kyoto 614

NETHERLANDS

Erikjan Bartelds, Duinoordsewed 1, Oostyoorne (Z.H.)

SWEDEN

Lars Åfeldt, c/o P-Club, Box 755, S-10130 Stockholm 1

SWITZERLAND

Vereinigung für Stotternde und Angehörige (VERSTA), Postfach 437, 8042 Zurich (Norman Bush)

UNITED STATES

National Stuttering Project, Robert Goldman, Box 33, Walnut Creek, California 94596
National Association of Councils of Stutterers, Michael Hartford, 1724 North Troy Street Nr. 772, Arlington, Virginia 22201

Glossary

This list of terms gives their meaning as associated with stammering or speech in general.

Some of the definitions below have been adapted from *Stuttering Words*, published by the Speech Foundation of America, to whom I express my thanks.

Anxiety A complex emotional state. In stammering, it is characterised by fear or dread of unpleasant events or unsatisfactory relationships caused by difficulty when speaking.

Approach-avoidance conflict This term describes the conflict which the stammerer experiences as he approaches a feared word or situation. His desire for avoidance of verbal difficulty vies for mastery with his desire for speaking; the conflict may be expressed outwardly by tension and struggle which interferes with speech.

Articulation The production of individual sounds in connected speech; or the movement of the speech organs in order to modify the stream of voiced or unvoiced air so that meaningful sounds are produced. The organs mainly involved are the jaw, lips, tongue and hard and soft palate.

Auditory feedback The sensations produced in the ears by one's own speech, either through airborne or bone-conducted vibrations.

Avoidance Anything the stammerer does in order to escape from stammering or evade having trouble while speaking. Avoidance may consist of keeping silent, changing words, using synonyms, coughing, pretending not to hear, etc.

Block or Blocking A moment of stammering referring to an instance when the speech muscles do not function properly; or to the stoppage or sensation of being 'stuck' experienced when the stammerer tries to talk and is temporarily prevented from speaking. To the stammerer it may be a moment of crisis which he has usually anticipated and that can, momentarily, interfere with ongoing speech.

Circumlocution A device used by stammerers to avoid feared words by rephrasing their thought using different words.

Consonant A speech sound made by complete or partial stoppage of the breath stream; there is touching or contact of two speech organs to modify the breath stream; broadly, any sound that is not a vowel.

Contact In speech, the touching of two speech organs in order to modify or change the breath (air) stream to produce a consonant sound. For example, the lips touch for 'b', 'p' and 'm'; the lower lip and upper teeth for 'f' and 'v'; the tip of the tongue touches the hard palate behind the upper teeth for 't', 'd', etc.

Covert Hidden, concealed, internal reactions or unobservable behaviour (as opposed to 'overt').

Delayed Auditory Feedback The speaker hears his own utterance slightly later than is usual – rather like an echo. This delay is usually created artificially by the use of a machine and, under laboratory or clinical conditions, the delay is approximately 0·1–0·2 seconds.

Disfluency   Refers to any sort of speech which is not smooth or fluent. All speakers talk disfluently at times – they hesitate or stumble to varying degrees. All stammerers are disfluent, but all disfluency is not stammering. This is particularly true for the disfluency noted in most small children.

Establishment   In stammering, the initial teaching of procedures or techniques to promote fluent speech.

Eye Contact   Looking the listener in the eye while talking to him. Generally a natural (although not a constant) interaction of the speaker's eyes with the eyes of the listener. Maintaining eye contact is considered important in stammering therapy to help the stammerer combat feelings of shame, embarrassment and avoidance.

Fear   To the stammerer, this is the anticipation of difficulty he may have when speaking. This fear of difficulty can vary from one person to another and may range from mild to very severe. It can, and sometimes does, paralyse thought and action. Some therapy is related to the amount of fear which is present. Stammering fears can be of situations or persons, of sounds or words, etc.

Feared Word   Refers to a word on which the stammerer anticipates he will have difficulty.

Fricative   A sound made by the airstream passing through such a narrow passage that audible, high-frequency currents are set up, for example 'f', 'v', 'th', etc. Certain high-frequency fricatives are also termed sibilants, for example 's', 'z', 'sh', etc.

Galvanic Skin Resistance/Response   Electrical resistance or response in the skin. The change in this resistance/response can be measured with a biofeedback machine (such as that produced by Alpha Ltd, Cambridge) and serves to help the stammerer to monitor his level of tension or relaxation. Sometimes used in therapy.

Group Therapy   Counselling or therapy structured in a group of between 3 and 9 stammerers. The interchange of feelings, ideas and discussion of stammering problems or the learning of a technique may be facilitated as the group member gains insight and understanding through a knowledge that others share his difficulties and that he is not alone with his problems.

Hard Palate   The bony, front part of the palate which forms the roof of the mouth.

Hypnosis   Artificially induced state similar in many respects to sleep, but characterised by extreme suggestibility and the continuance of rapport between client and hypnotist.

Inferiority Complex   There are many different definitions of this term. A general description would be: a pattern of emotionally influenced ideas concerning what a person feels to be his own inferiority; strong and generalised feelings of being inferior and inadequate tend to prevent the person's ability to achieve his full potential. An acute sense of inferiority may result either in timidity or, through over-compensation, in exaggerated aggressiveness.

Initiation or Initiating In speech, the beginning or starting of a sound, syllable or word; or the commencement of speech.

Light Contacts Loose or tension-free contacts or touching of the speech organs in the production of consonant sounds, especially plosive sounds such as 't', 'd', 'p', 'b', 'k', and 'g'. In therapy, the client may be helped to make these contacts loose and easy as opposed to the hard, tense contacts which occur in stammering.

Maintenance The continued use of fluent and/or controlled speech after regular therapy has ended.

Masking The complete obscuring of one tone or sounds by another. Interference with the normal hearing process by simultaneously presenting another sound of a different frequency, intensity, quality or pattern in one or both ears. Such a masking sound may be channelled through headphones or ear-pieces so that the stammerer cannot hear himself speak. If the masking sound is of sufficient loudness, many stammerers will become more fluent.

Mirror Practice Self-analysis or observation through mirror practice; working on reading or speaking in front of a mirror so that the stammerer can observe what he does when stammering and find ways to modify, change or eliminate habitual stammering behaviour.

Modifying the Stammering Pattern Changing recurring patterns which are noted when the stammer occurs. Therapists may suggest that the client can and should change his stammering behaviour and learn to stammer in different, easier and more appropriate ways. In so changing and modifying his stammering pattern, he learns that he can change his way of speaking and stammering and that he can develop a style of talking which is less abnormal and free of excessive tension and struggle.

Non-fluency See **Disfluency**

Objective Attitude The attitude that is desirable for the stammerer to have towards his stammering; a feeling relatively independent of personal prejudice or apprehensions and not distorted by shame and embarrassment; the acceptance of stammering as a problem rather than a curse or an affliction.

Obsession A persistent or recurrent preoccupation with an idea or feeling which is often irrational or unreasonable; the preoccupation of some stammerers with their problem may, in some cases, be regarded as obsessional.

Overt Open, outward, visible or audible stammering behaviour (as opposed to 'covert').

Parent Counselling This involves establishing a relationship between parent(s) and therapist to enable the latter to help and advise on the feelings, habits and policies of the parents as regards their child, so as to diminish parental feelings of anxiety, guilt, annoyance and so on and assist in devising appropriate ways of interacting with and handling the child and his speech. Since parental attitudes can sometimes aggravate disfluent speech and a healthy attitude in the home is an aid to therapy, wise and sympathetic parental counselling is frequently thought to be important.

Plosive Any speech sound made by stopping the airstream momentarily and then suddenly releasing it, as with 'p', 'b', 't', 'd', 'k', and 'g'.

Positive Emotion The predominantly sympathetic responses of a person to the circumstances or people who surround him. It encompasses terms like hope, pleasure, joy, and so on. Within limits, positive emotion is thought to facilitate the fluency of speech.

Postponement Devices Many stammerers when anticipating difficulty in speech try to put off saying the feared sound or word. Various devices may be used to postpone speaking the feared word such as inserting extra words, sounds or phrases or repeating previously spoken words.

Prolongation This term can refer to stammering behaviour when the speaker finds he is continuing on a sound longer than he wishes, e.g. fffffffather or mmmmmmother. Prolongation may also mean the deliberate elongation of speech sounds as part of a fluency-shaping technique to help the stammerer modify his stammering pattern and acquire greater flow and ease when speaking

Psychotherapy The treatment of behavioural or emotional problems by counselling, or by re-educating and influencing the person's mental approaches and his ways of thinking, or of evaluating his problems; any procedures intended to improve the condition of a person that are directed at a change in his mental approach to his problems, particularly his attitude towards himself and his environment. The amount of psychotherapy that is advisable in adult stammering therapy must depend on the needs of each client, his type of stammer and the views of the therapist regarding treatment.

Secondary Symptoms Abnormal or unusual actions or movements exhibited by a stammerer when trying to talk. These include eye blinking, eye closure, grimaces, hand clenching, foot tapping, scratching the face, etc. These movements have become an integral part of the stammer and tend to help in its continuance. The modification of these movements tends to weaken the stammer.

Soft Palate The soft, muscular fold of skin which is suspended from the back of the hard palate.

Starter Any trick or device which the stammerer uses in order to help him start speaking when he anticipates or experiences a stammer. These starting devices may include head jerking, coughing, insertion of sounds such as 'er' or 'm', etc.

Stammering Pattern The specific things that a person does and the order in which he does them that interfere with his speaking and constitute his overt stammer.

Substitutions The changing of words when stammering is anticipated or the use of synonyms.

Time Pressure At the moment that he is expected or wants to speak, or during speech, the stammerer may believe that the listener(s) is becoming impatient or bored and so he may experience feelings of panic, haste or urgency. He feels under 'time pressure' and with no time to lose, and therefore has a strong need to speak instantly or to rush through the utterance with great speed. A basic feature of stammering behaviour is that the majority of stammerers feel under time pressure to a greater or lesser extent much of the time that they are speaking or about to speak.

Utterance   The act of speaking; the expression of thoughts through the use of words.

Vocalisation   The act or method of producing voice for speech. We breathe air into our lungs and, if we are speaking, as this air is breathed out it passes through the larynx in the throat. In the larynx are the vocal cords consisting of two folds of skin, which may be open, closed or vibrating. When we hold our breath, the cords are closed or together and the breath is constricted under them; the cords may be closed during a severe block. When we speak, the breath stream activates the vocal cords so that they vibrate and produce voice or vocalisation.

Voiced   Sounds spoken with voice because the vocal cords are vibrating; all vowel sounds ('a', 'e', 'i', 'o', and 'u') are voiced, and some consonants, for example 'b', 'd', 'g', 'z', and 'l'.

LIBRARY
NURSE EDUCATION CENTRE
BRIDGEND GENERAL

Index

LIBRARY
NURSE EDUCATION CENTRE
BRIDGEND GENERAL